TAKING CONTROL
TOGETHER

Real Life Stories on Caring for Yourself and a Loved One
With Multiple Sclerosis

By Jillian Kingsford Smith

Taking Control Together: Real Life Stories on Caring for Yourself and a Loved One With Multiple Sclerosis

Copyright © 2015 Jillian Kingsford Smith
1st published 2015 by Take20 Stories, Brisbane Qld Australia
www.take20stories.com

Liability Disclaimer: The material contained in this book is general in nature and does not represent professional advice. It is not intended to provide specific guidance for particular circumstances and it should not be relied on as a basis for any decisions to take action on any matter that it covers. Readers should obtain professional advice before acting on any information in this book. Neither the Author nor the Publisher can be held responsible for any loss or claim arising out of the use, or misuse, of the suggestions made or the failure to take medical advice.

National Library of Australia Cataloguing-in-publication data:

Author:	Kingsford-Smith, Jillian, author.
Title:	Taking control : a collection of inspiring stories for people living with multiple sclerosis / by Jillian Kingsford Smith.
ISBN:	9780987537522 (paperback)
Subjects:	Multiple sclerosis--Australia--Patients--Interviews.
	Multiple sclerosis--Australia--Patients--Family relationships
	Caregivers--Interviews.
	Care of the sick.

Dewey Number: 362.196834

Cover Design: Vanessa Maynard.

DEDICATION

For my family. Always and forever.

"Some people care too much. I think it's called love."

- A.A. Milne, Winnie-the-Pooh

CONTENTS

INTRODUCTION

by Jillian Kingsford Smith

....

Nothing tests the expression 'in sickness and in health' quite like a chronic illness. Living with a condition such as multiple sclerosis can take a toll on even the best relationship; the person who's sick may not feel the way he or she did before the illness and the person who's not sick may not know how to handle the changes. The strain may push both people to breaking point.

Trapped, lonely, out of control, helpless, guilt, anger, frustration and bewilderment are just some of the emotions that people continually mentioned throughout this book. But with every negative emotion came an avalanche of positive character traits. Gratitude, resilience, empathy, vision, inner strength, friendship, unconditional love and benevolence are just a few.

About two and a half years ago – April Fool's Day 2012 to be exact – I was diagnosed with MS. It was a shock and quite unexpected and has brought many changes and challenges. But one of the best things I've done in that time is write "Taking Control: A Collection of Inspiring Stories for People Living with MS." The book was released in May of 2013 and quickly became a best seller. It is a collection of 15 people talking about their own journey with MS.

Throughout the process of writing this first book I identified that the caregivers or supporters of those with MS didn't have anyone to turn to for individualised support. There is so little information out there for people actually living with MS but there is even less information for those who are the support network. This may include a spouse, parent, child, friend or even the professional caregiver.

A chronic or long-term illness – such as multiple sclerosis – and its treatment poses special problems. Most of these issues are obvious and well documented. Both the patient and the supporter need to learn how to live with the physical effects of the illness, manage treatments and specialists and try to maintain some semblance of emotional balance and positive self-image on top of this.

And it doesn't end there. As well as needing to find ways to deal with the stress involved with chronic illness, everyone in the support network will also need to maintain trust and confidence in the doctors, especially when recovery isn't always possible; know how to deal with flares in the symptoms and critically maintain social relationships despite facing an uncertain medical future or unpredictable symptoms. In fact, every person interviewed strongly counsels that avoiding social isolation is a key factor in managing a chronic illness.

Caregiving can be emotionally taxing and physically draining. Recent studies across Australia, America and Europe all cite that carers have the lowest wellbeing of any large group and are at least 40 per cent more likely to also suffer from a chronic health condition themselves.

As a result, caregiver health is quickly becoming a public health issue that requires more focused attention from health professionals, policy makers and caregivers to ensure the health and safety of those individuals dedicating their lives to the care of others. Increasing appropriate mental health services and medical care for family caregivers are important steps toward addressing caregiver health.

But as the stories in this book illustrate, providing support for a loved one with a chronic illness can also bring a tremendous amount of opportunity and fulfilment. It's undeniable that being diagnosed with a chronic illness is a game changer, but everyone interviewed for 'Taking Control Together' has proven that dire situations can inspire positive changes. The journey's described in this book are a testament to the prevailing human spirit, where we witness people often digging deep to find an inner strength they didn't know they possessed.

My own family inspired me to write 'Taking Control Together.' I wanted to create a resource that would help them. We've always believed that story telling is the best medium for learning and finding comfort. Through the process of writing my first book I was amazed and encouraged by the untold stories of the supporters acting behind-the-scenes. They often bear everything that we do in living with a chronic illness and more.

And as with the first book, I found a pattern repeating. As I approached (and sometimes stalked) people I wanted to interview, these people would universally say "I'm happy to share my story but there's nothing special about me," or "I can't imagine why anyone would find me interesting."

But interviewing these people was unlike anything else I've ever experienced as a writer. Many had never given themselves an opportunity, let alone permission, to speak so frankly about the battles they face, the frustrations and fears they deal with or the triumphs they have achieved. The stories within are an outpouring of emotion but also a celebration of the good times. Just like the person living with the chronic illness, they have had good days and bad – and they very openly share those details. You will be moved by their own stories because you'll be able to relate – whether you're living with an illness or providing care. And in relating, you'll be able to take comfort that life does go on... And maybe – just as it has for everyone in this book – it turns into something even better than what you had before.

STEPHANIE MILLS

*"If I was the one in the public eye I would find it a tremendous
pressure to have a condition that people might identify with;
they look to you for inspiration or support and all you're trying to do
is make it through the day."*

**Canadian-born Stephanie Mills moved to Australia several years ago to
pursue post-graduate studies and further her career in the entertainment industry. She has excelled in her career and also found love along
the way, marrying the well-known Australian comedian Tim Ferguson.**

I met Tim in 2007 at the Australian International Movie
Convention on the Gold Coast. We were both there for work;
I was a delegate of the company I was working for and Tim was
hosting the event. I had seen him around the event all week but it
wasn't until the final night of the convention that we started talking.
Earlier in the evening he had made a funny comment to one of my
colleagues that she had found quite offensive and I decided I needed
to approach him about the remark on her behalf – armed with the
courage of a few sauv blancs, of course.

So after the dinner event I walked up to Tim and proceeded to give
him a serve.

"I don't know who you are but you made a joke that insulted my
colleague. If you're as good a comedian as everyone says, surely you
could have come up with a better joke." There was a certain amount

of truth in the statement. I didn't know who Tim was, as I'd only been working in Australia a short time.

He just sat there smiling; waiting until I'd finished my rant and simply asked "Where are you from?"

"Canada," I replied. And from that moment on we talked and talked and haven't stopped. That particular night we talked through until 6am the next day. We talked about life and philosophy and feminism; all the topics I hadn't talked deeply about since my university days.

I checked my watch for the first time in hours and realised what time it was.

"I've got a flight to catch. I've got to get moving," I said.

"You're not going back to Canada today are you?" questioned Tim.

"No. I live in Australia now; Melbourne, in fact." As the conversation unfolded we realised we lived within a few streets of each other. Tim wanted to see me again, so we swapped details and as they say, 'that was that!' He actually called me as I was passing through security at the Gold Coast airport for my return flight home. We became inseparable.

On that very first night Tim admitted to me that he had MS. He hadn't yet gone public with the news and I guess because I didn't really understand who he was and how recognisable he is in Australia, I didn't realise the full significance of what he was telling me.

He was very up-front about his diagnosis from the beginning because he believed that we had something special together and wanted to lay all the cards on the table as early as possible. I wasn't particularly phased by the announcement though. I have a cousin in Canada with MS and whenever I looked at Tim he seemed fine. He was walking normally and didn't have any physical signs of being unwell. We had such a strong connection immediately and it was great to have everything out in the open.

Despite growing up with a family member with MS, I had no perception of how the disease progresses. My cousin – to this day

— has no physical signs of MS, so I had no reference for what the disease might involve for Tim. It wasn't until about three or four months later, when he had a bit of an episode that compromised his balance and mobility, that I started to think how this might affect us; particularly when the symptoms were becoming more noticeable. I started researching things a little more and focussing on what it might mean for us. But really I just dealt with it the same way that I prepare for most things in life. It made more sense for me to remain calm and rational so that I could work out what we might be facing and how we would deal with that.

There's only been one episode that has really rattled me and that was when his mobility issues progressed to the point where he needed a stick all the time. And it wasn't actually the introduction of a constant walking aid that concerned me. It was more the fact that Tim hadn't yet gone public with his condition so we both had to cover it up. People would recognise him and then see the stick but instead of asking Tim, they'd approach me to ask what was wrong. I found it quite offensive and also extremely confronting. I never knew what to say. It didn't help that Tim would constantly change his story as to why he was using a stick - ever bringing humour to the situation.

I legitimately didn't know what to say though. Sometimes I would make jokes as well, other times I'd use his standard and plausible reason (he fell off a horse, he hurt his leg, etc.). But if I was in a bit of a mood I'd do my 'Will & Grace' routine, which is a parody of the sharp-witted Karen Walker.

"What's wrong with Tim's leg? Why does he have a stick?" they'd ask.

"What stick?" I'd reply. "I don't see a stick, honey."

It would invariably close the conversation down. Although I'll admit it wasn't often that I'd hold a straight face to deliver that zinger!

It was during the time Tim first started using his stick more in public that I found the hardest. It wasn't because he was harder to care for. It was simply the burden of helping him keep his secret. I wanted to do everything I could to protect him. Tim's best friend Mark and I both debated with him at different times how much easier it would be if the public knew. I sensed the dread Tim was feeling on those days he was performing a gig and didn't feel a hundred per cent. He takes tremendous pride in what he does and would hate to think he was letting anyone down. Particularly if he was hosting an event, he preferred the audience didn't see him on his walking stick. But after a few falls and perhaps even his own reconciliation with the situation, the stick became a permanent companion. It was around this time that Mark finally talked Tim across the line and he went public with the news. Mark's rationale to Tim was that hiding the condition was only wasting energy and it would continue to get harder; plus, what did he have to lose in telling the truth?

Despite his eventual agreement with Mark, the public announcement wasn't planned. As it happened, Tim was being interviewed by a journalist he trusted and the question about the stick was brought up and he answered truthfully for once. He called me straight after the interview to tell me what he'd done. We were both so excited and even celebrated that night. I was happy and relieved. Strangely, all these years later we still get asked about the stick but now we get to choose whether we answer truthfully or comically. The pressure to hide has disappeared. And you know, the things he was worried would happen when he revealed his diagnosis never eventuated.

If I was the one in the public eye I would find it a tremendous pressure to have a condition that people might identify with; they look to you for inspiration or support and all you're trying to do is make it through the day.

Tim doesn't want to be defined by his MS. He doesn't want that to be the only topic of conversation. Naturally he has many people approach him to ask questions about MS but I still get my fair share that walk up to me rather than Tim. I think they believe it's more polite or discreet to bypass Tim and pull me aside to ask questions! I understand that nine times out of ten, people are asking from concern but I have little patience for it. I've gotten very good at discerning between people who are genuinely fond of Tim and those who are just being nosy. It constantly amazes me that people will blatantly ask quite personal things, such as his treatment protocol or how he manages things at home. Mostly I provide a canned response of 'yep, we're doing great. Everything is just fine.' I remain fairly vague in those situations and frankly the nosiness is boring.

I don't try to hide my private life but despite – or perhaps because of – being married to a public figure I'm not very forthcoming with many details. I have kept my maiden name and even at work (and remember I work for an entertainment company) it took people over a year to figure out exactly who my husband is. The discretion has allowed me to remain my own person in professional circles; defined by my own ability and characteristics rather than by a well-known figure with a disability.

And we also surround ourselves with supportive but down-to-earth friends so I've never felt frustrated or that I'm losing my sense of self. They're the type of people who know that if we need help we'll ask; otherwise they're just around being great friends. In fact, amongst our close circle of friends, the only times the disability thing ever comes up is if we're planning on going out for dinner and we have a brief discussion about the venues with the best accessibility.

I think we've conditioned our friends and family to a certain extent as to what kind of help we need and when we just need the company and friendship more so than any kind of structured support. And to a large degree I think this has also helped me retain my sense of self. By being more open about everything, people don't feel a need to constantly talk to me about the MS or offer assistance when it's not needed. The MS only becomes relevant when we need it to. I'm not consumed by it or continually confronted by it from every corner. I've realised that being quite open with our closest friends can only be beneficial. I use the expression 'we will make every effort' quite liberally! It helps to frame our social life and also removes any pressure of being somewhere at a certain time. People now under-stand that we genuinely try to and want to participate in the things we commit to but it's not always possible. Things happen. The MS can unexpectedly take things out of our control. But the flexibility we both practice allows us to live a life less stressful.

In 2010 I had surgery on my back and since then I've had some issues being able to physically help Tim as much as I'd like. Tim's a tall guy and although certainly not heavy I am limited now in what I can lift. It wasn't as much of an issue immediately after my surgery because Tim was still predominantly using his walking stick, but five years later he's using the wheel chair more frequently and I struggle pulling the chair in and out of vehicles or managing the chair on uneven and sloping sidewalks. It really is only occasionally that I worry about how much I struggle but also highlights how some of the things we might consider so simple can quickly become difficult.

And I always underestimate the amount of time it takes to do things. I forget about it until we actually venture out and then I realise how much more difficult it is to open doors and manoeuvre Tim and his chair, or get into the car or a taxi. When I plan things, in my mind I think we can be somewhere in 5 minutes but the reality is that it takes 20 minutes longer. It never stops us from doing things but it's a lesson I still need to have ingrained I guess – to allow more time to get from A to B! I'm not an impatient person but I have a real issue being late to appointments or keeping people waiting – so something has to give; either my attitude or the execution of logistics. And at the end of the day, none of this is life changing stuff. It's just a matter of appropriate planning.

When one area of your life is a bit out of control – and for us it's the MS – I've found it's really important to try and keep everything else stable. Not long ago Tim had a bad MS episode and at the same time the company I work for was restructuring and I ended up being offered a new role. We had moved from Melbourne to Sydney for me to join this company a few months before, but the restructure and subsequent promotion all happened very quickly. The state of flux threw me a bit and I felt quite panicked about life for a while. It made me realise how vulnerable we actually were. We had never taken advantage of any home care services and to be honest, we hadn't even gotten referred to a neurologist or even a GP after we'd moved cities. In fact there were dozens of things we hadn't done after our interstate move, and in hindsight, we should have paid more attention to building that safety net around us a bit earlier so that when life became unbalanced we didn't both lose our sense of stability. It was the first time and the only time I felt that I couldn't care for Tim on my own. I needed to establish the safety net.

In these times of instability you realise how well you can actually cope and get on with life when everything in your personal universe isn't lining up. Life is never going to stop throwing curve balls at you but I think trying to minimise unnecessary disruption is a great skill to learn for both the person living with MS and their support network.

In my mind, a good safety net needs to have the following components:

- A medical team you can trust and that resonates with you: Obviously this would include a neurologist, a GP and hospital system you're comfortable in.
- An occupational therapist: A consultation with an occupational therapist can be confronting but the strategies they'll suggest are intended to make life easier.
- And access to an MS nurse, coordinator or social worker can also be handy.

I think we get so involved in the clinical side of MS that we forget there's quite a few resources intended to make our life a bit easier, from subsidies for cooling devices and access to cheaper taxis and transportation through to home help. Unfortunately, there's no single place to find all this information but a good place to start is with the services coordinators at any of the multiple sclerosis organisations around the world. It can be daunting to coordinate all this additional information and even knowing what to ask is complex.

And a word of caution with all these professionals: It is completely appropriate for you to push back; to ask questions and to question their advice. I've come to recognise that the advice the specialists give is often worst-case scenario and they will lay out the future risk we may have to contend with. So where possible, try to step back and examine the information being given to you. Maybe categorise the information into time frames. For example, is this something I need to worry about now? Is doom imminent? Or perhaps this is just something unappealing that I may have to prepare for in the future? We can be certain that there are few certainties when it comes to MS.

I've found that disability – at least in Australia – is also quite standardised. I'll explain what I mean. Tim is self-employed. He works constantly, but he essentially works for himself. Whenever we've sought assistance from various agencies for support they've been unable to wrap their mind around how self-employed people operate. I've found that the questions we were being asked to qualify us for assistance were framed around 'normal' work situations. 'How many office hours do you work?' 'How is your office set up for mobility and to address your mobility?' 'What salary do you take home every fortnight?'

Self-employment is a fantastic thing for people with MS as it means they can work flexibly to suit their energy or mobility. Yet the very benevolent systems designed to support people with a disability make it very difficult to access assistance when self-employed. Determining the appropriate assistance you might qualify for and then navigating the enormous amount of paperwork, medical signoffs and permissions has been difficult and complex. So much so that it seemed easier to give up at times. Having said that, an experienced social worker, disabilities coordinator or even an employment solicitor can greatly assist you in understanding any services, legal rights or even employment and financial implications.

Most people fail to realise that with the diagnosis of MS (or any chronic illness) it's not just the person being diagnosed who has to live with the condition but it's also the support network around them. Everyone plays a unique and important role. My life has changed significantly and, I imagine, will continue to over time.

On a personal level I rarely sleep through the night any longer. This is something that very few people would ever highlight when they talk about living with MS. But because Tim is often unsettled at night, I am too. I've adjusted to waking up frequently throughout the night, but I'm sure it's not healthy for either of us to sustain.

As an entertainer, Tim has never worked regular hours and I find myself being hyper-aware of his need to rest. I want to ensure that he doesn't push himself too hard. Perhaps I come across a bit controlling at times, especially when I insist on him taking time out. He's a very motivated person and always wants to go above and beyond so I do feel it my duty to monitor him and be the voice of reason if he's over-committing. I recognise the patterns now. If he travels with gigs for a week and then comes back for a week of teaching then I know it's imperative for him to keep a good week or so clear after that to recover. Someone's got to be the planner or the gatekeeper on this stuff.

And the funniest thing of all is that I hate planning. I hate cleaning and cooking and planning everything we need to do to keep our life in order. I love Tim and our life together and of course I'd do anything to make life comfortable but I really do hate planning!

So our work-around is that we get a cleaner in to take care of the house every fortnight. It might seem like a luxury to some, but as I work full time with long hours, it conserves my own energy to focus on what really matters. It's funny how we consider small things like this a luxury when really it's a necessity. I don't understand why so many people feel such guilt at getting help around the house.

Tim is incredibly good at looking after me. He keeps me very grounded. It may only sound like a little thing but I love that every morning he gets up, makes me a coffee and brings it to me in bed. Even though I can hear him bumping furniture, clanging cups and muttering swearwords the entire time, I love that it's our ritual. It's clearly his way of making sure my own day gets off to a great start. And it is a big deal to me. Have you ever watched someone trying to balance a cup of coffee on their walker from the kitchen to the bedroom? It's nerve racking!

He's also conscious of my own energy. If he knows I've had a huge day at work he'll look after dinner. It may just be defrosting something to go straight into the oven but he's planning ahead and being mindful. It's his version of 'making dinner.'

And he's never once demanded my time or attention either. If I've planned a night out with girlfriends he wouldn't dream of interfering with that, no matter how poorly he felt. Again, he's conscious of my time during the work week and I guess also my need to have time out with friends. I think it's very important for the support person or primary caregiver to have their own outlet from the disease.

One of our greatest advantages is that we're a communicative couple. We discuss everything and are very open so there's never any subtext or issues left unspoken. And part of that equation is also just being in tune with each other emotionally, so some things don't even need to be discussed.

There are days when I just don't physically feel like pushing a wheel chair. Early on I felt a bit guilty about my attitude but as his mobility changed and the chair became a more regular item in our lives, I got my guilt. Because it's not about guilt. If the tables were turned and Tim had to take greater physical care of me then I'd be devastated if he didn't tell me when he didn't feel like pushing a chair or whatever the issue may be. That dynamic of complete honesty has been very important to us. If we didn't have that then neither of us could protect our wellbeing and I also fear that we might consider one or the other a burden. At the end of the day we're human and it's going to be natural to feel frustration or anger or exhaustion. Allow yourself to feel the emotions because bottling it up helps no one. The role of care giver does not mean you have to be everything to everyone all the time. That's an unrealistic notion.

Tim is very good at separating his condition from himself. He's always been this way throughout our relationship and we have amazing chemistry because of it. I know Tim for the person he is without MS, despite the fact he's lived with the condition for so long. But just as importantly, I think he is assured of the person he is without MS. In times when I get frustrated with things – say the wheelchair not doing what it should – Tim understands that I'm not cranky with him. I'm cranky at a piece of equipment. He never pulls the 'but I've got MS' excuse either. He'll sometimes make excuses that things don't get done because he's a 'creative,' but he'll never pull the pity card.

I recognise how important it is for a caregiver to take care of themselves but I must admit, I don't take care of myself as well as I should. But that has less to do with being consumed with caring for Tim and everything to do with being a little bit lazy. I know the value of eating healthy food and exercising but if I was being honest then I'd admit I really like eating chips and watching TV!

And while I joke about not looking after myself, I think I have worked hard at making sure my life (and I guess Tim's for that matter) is not all about me being in the primary care-giver's role and it's not about MS every day. I can't stress the importance of this enough. It's been really important for me to be able to leave MS at the door when I enter my office. It's not that it ceases to exist but I'm simply not consumed by it and can focus on my job, which I also enjoy tremendously. And because I'm focusing on doing the best job that I can do it provides me with my own sense of identity and self-worth.

On the flip side, when I leave the office I make a deliberate effort to leave my work there so as I can be emotionally and mentally present when I'm at home. I'm usually successful at this and stick by my rules that the weekends are for Tim and I.

Life is always full of compromises and we've certainly learned the art of compromise whilst living with MS. Sometimes the smallest things are the things you notice the most. It's funny how you can become very clinical and precise about the big, scary medical stuff, but it's the small things that intrude on your lifestyle that you notice the most.

I know this sounds petty but my life is full of constant clutter. It's not an inconvenience, but merely an observation. The ramps and handrails around the house are a constant reminder. As young people it's not something you contemplate needing to live with.

Sometimes I see other residential properties advertised and think to myself how nice they'd be, but then I'll see that there are too many stairs or the wheelchair access is poor so I quickly dismiss the property, knowing that they'd be unsuitable in the long term. I don't necessarily see it as a sacrifice but rather that we have narrower options than other people. I guess our needs are vastly different to other home-owners. Our life isn't better or worse than anyone else's; our reality is just different.

We try to go back to Canada once a year to visit my family and with travel come a new set of challenges. Believe it or not the logistics are actually easier now that Tim uses his chair more. We've been so lucky that every airport we've had to transit between has been very accommodating to people in wheelchairs. But the airlines still seem to have a whacky habit of destroying every mobility device we've ever owned. I truly believe the baggage handlers look at each individual device and try to work out how to damage it the most. It's like some sort of sick game of dare. I've written letters over and over to the airlines after they've damaged something, reminding them that they basically need to consider mobility devices as people's legs and take the greatest care; to no avail however. Maybe one day!

I love going home to visit my family. It's great to have someone dote on us for a few weeks. And travel still remains a great joy for both of us. We're mindful of the time of year we choose to travel and that we also need to allow more time for transit and recovery because it can be exhausting, but once we're at the destination it's just magic. That is one of the other compromises I've had to make; I love Canada in the summer but I know that if Tim is with me it's not going to work. He's just too sensitive to the heat and humidity. I really try to find the joy in Canadian winters but I've got a lot of work to do where that's concerned!

Someone asked me if anything scares me about my future with Tim – and I guess more specifically, the fact that Tim has MS.

I guess the answer is 'no'. I worry about him when I'm travelling for work, or late coming home, but ultimately, I'm not scared for our future. To be honest though, I never think too far ahead in life. I'm not burying my head in the sand but we tend to both live in the moment. If either of us wants to do something then we work out how to do it now. 'Some day' is not an expression used very often in our home. As opportunities arise we take advantage of them. And I'm not suggesting that we live irresponsibly either but we just don't put stuff off.

There are greater things about the future that scare me than MS. And they're probably the same things that anyone else might be scared about. About losing your job. About having an accident. About the wellbeing of your family. Tim's health could go downhill rapidly tomorrow but I can't change that. For now it's about being rational and prepared for what we can control. It's a very grown up thing to feel. And I know I can count on Tim to tell me realistically how he's feeling and we'll deal with it then. But until that point our focus is about just getting on and living life to the fullest; and what a great life it is.

Dear Stephanie

Together we get a lot done, and none of what I do would be possible without you. For starters, you make me feel the impossible is doable, and we can achieve it together. Plus, I wouldn't be able to get out of the house without your help, and certainly never on time!

Quite often, it's the little things that make getting the big things done a tricky business. This is where it's always good to know we are sharing the annoyances. MS has a hundred different faces for everybody. But for me it means I move that little bit more slowly. I'm quite effective once I arrive, but it does mean we have to plan things more carefully. And because I'm male, my planning techniques are completely woeful, so the natural ability that you transfer from your professional life to our private life is invaluable.

We spend a lot of time together and I love being in your orbit. You are my favourite company in the world. We always laugh, we enjoy the same projects, the same movies, all the same pastimes. When it comes to socialising, we do it well together and we do it well separately. And this is important because the weight of MS has the potential to turn us into home bodies. However working in the entertainment industry means that we have to be social, so sometimes the parties are work but they do play an important function in the way that we live together. You are the best party date – beautiful and fascinating.

I used to apologise for MS a lot. But I try not to do that anymore. Apologising actually just places the burden of forgiving onto the other person. And really it's just best when we both accept that MS is a factor in our lives and it has to be dealt with; we almost treat MS like a third person in our family. We make sure neither of us is to blame if we get frustrated, angry or held up with the challenges that MS brings.

You've helped some couples face their MS diagnosis and I am so proud of you for that. Your first-hand experience as the wife of someone with MS gives your advice insight and emotional affinity. And your 'Canadian calm' is a wonder.

But the main thing is that we have a lot of fun. You're enormously successful in your work and I just try as hard as I can to match your abilities. And then at home we love each other's company and I'm just crazy about you. It's cheeky being a couple the way we are because we can show off in front of all the other couples and show them how much fun we have.

I couldn't get anything done or be able to bravely think ahead if you weren't in my life. You helped me climb out of the hole I found myself in whilst dealing with MS solo. My life without you would be far more nomadic and I simply wouldn't have any grounding or roots and I'd be ever going around in circles.

Now all my circles lead back to you, and love is all around.

Tim

EMMA BALFOUR - DAUGHTER

"A very small part of me is waiting for that first sign of MS to show up, but then on the other hand I think 'so what?' At the end of the day there's very little I can do about it and whatever happens will happen. I can't expend too much precious energy tying myself in knots over it. I always come back to making the most of what's happening in my life now."

Having travelled for 20 years as one of the world's most recognised models, Emma Balfour once again calls Sydney home. It is here she raises her two sons with her partner Andrew whilst being the 'dutiful daughter' to her mother and father, both diagnosed with MS. Her relationship with each of her parents is both unique and complex based on their different reactions and needs as to how they live with MS, as is the perspective that living with the disease has brought to how she wants to live her own life.

***

I was born in Sydney and both of my parents lived in a boatshed on Louisa Road in Balmain. They would recount stories about how they used to lower me down to the water's edge in a basket. Back then the area was dotted with shipbuilding yards and my parents often wonder if there weren't some environmental hazard from the heavy metals in the area that contributed to them both being diagnosed with MS within a few years of each other. There was a park close by and it was off-limits to play in as apparently it was contaminated in some way. Still today, Dad more than Mum ponders the significance of the metal contamination that heavy industry brought to the neighbourhood, but he's just searching for answers.

When I was about 18 months old we all moved back to Adelaide and that's where I really grew up. My little brother was born a few years after we moved to Adelaide but Mum and Dad ended up getting divorced about two years after that. I was about six years old, Mum was 26 and Dad was 35. I look at old photos of my parents and they were a fabulous looking couple but now that I'm older and know their individual personalities I can't fathom how they ever got together!

I left home at 16 and moved to London at 18 for my modelling career and to be honest it's a little difficult to fully piece together my parent's diagnosis because I was living overseas and away from all the day-to-day drama. But I do remember that when I was about 21, Dad telephoned me from hospital. I think he'd just been hospitalised for his first MS episode. His speech was slurred and he was clearly a bit distraught but trying to reassure me that everything was okay.

"It's all going to be alright Emma," he said through his tears. "I haven't had a stroke; I don't have a brain tumour. They don't really know what it is, but it's all going to be fine. I'm getting better and I just don't want you to worry at all." I was sitting on my bed 10,000 miles away in London and wandering what the fuck was going on.

I'd never seen or heard my Dad cry before, so it was all quite alarming. He was also clearly terrified, but what could I do? At the time, my brother was about 15 and living with him. Within a few months of this first episode they both travelled to London to visit me and I couldn't tell that anything was wrong with Dad. Whatever had happened before seemed to have fixed itself. With the wisdom of hindsight we can now label the hospitalisation as Dad's first episode, but 25 years or so back, MS was a difficult disease to diagnose. I know he experienced another episode again after his trip to the UK, but I didn't find out about this until many years later.

My modelling career had really taken off but I'd get back to Australia once or twice a year and the progression of his MS at that point wasn't very obvious. His walking was a little bit slower and getting around was just a little bit more difficult. But Dad was still Dad. I'm sure he was trying to hide from me just how bad his symptoms were actually becoming, but like a lot of men, he decided to completely ignore the whole thing, thinking it was bullshit. He didn't let it invade his world, at least not publicly. We've had many strong words over the years about him ignoring the blatant facts but his standard response is that it's his way of soldiering on.

Once I moved back to Australia in 1998 he seemed to slow down a bit. Or maybe I just noticed it more because I was seeing him more often. His health was certainly part of the reason I decided to come back to Australia and he was becoming less portable and just 'older' in general. He was about 50 when he finally received a confirmed diagnosis of MS.

My relationship with Dad – as with Mum – has certainly had its ups and downs, but I'm still terribly close to him. I'm much closer to him as an adult than I was as a child. Maybe it's because I lived with Mum after the divorce.

I didn't know a lot about MS. I had heard of it – growing up in a time where every kid in Australia participated in the MS Read-a-thons – but I thought it was a young person's disease. I asked Dad a million questions and I certainly didn't expect my Dad to be dealing with MS later in his life. He talked me through how the brain worked and what MS was doing to his own brain, but I was more interested in how the disease would affect him as a whole and what treatments would be best for him. I guess I just wanted to know what the prognosis was going to be because when you first hear about MS you think it's going to be an incredibly rapid and degenerative disease - which mostly it's not. But it's easy to think the worst when you first find out someone has MS. Dad's own progression was so slow but still noticeable.

He's done every test and consultation under the sun and each and every time ended up with a different set of variables. It's all just so goddamn unpredictable. I can't describe how annoying the exercise of monitoring – let alone treating – MS can be. To be honest I think I find it more frustrating than Dad does. I think Dad has become resigned to the downward decline that seems to be unfolding. He may be resigned to what the MS is doing to him but I can tell he's still depressed about it, and that doesn't help. Quite a few years back he went to a retreat at the Gawler Foundation and he came back bouncing off the walls. He was so excited and positive and made many of the changes that the retreat recommended, including adopting a vegan diet. But after doing all that and shifting his attitude he eventually went back to his old ways. I imagine he expected the results to be bigger and when they weren't, it was easier to revert to a mindset that was habitual. I can understand what he went through. He pinned all his hopes to a certain protocol and when he didn't get the results he so desperately wanted, he felt like he was back to square one. That has to be frustrating. He has stuck with the vegan diet however and this surely has to be beneficial.

Whenever Dad goes for a new test or treatment I mimic his hope, but at the same time I've learned to be realistic. There are massive changes that could be made in my father's life that would improve his situation. And they're not all medical. I think half the battle is getting himself into a healthy and happier mental place in life. And until he makes those changes and starts eliminating stress from his life his MS is going to be unstable. I really believe that how you're feeling emotionally or mentally is going to affect how you're feeling physically.

A resilient and positive mindset is certainly not to be underestimated. When things are going well, his body doesn't behave like a rigid piece of wood – which is one of the MS symptoms. But the minute he gets stressed he just goes stiff. He simply can't do anything. So if that isn't a metaphor for everything, then I don't know what is. But it is a bit of a battle to get him to see what I see. I just want better things for my Dad; not just on the MS side of things but for his life as a whole.

As both of my parents grow older it's getting harder to distinguish what is the MS progressing and what is simply the effects of old age. Perhaps the age thing is compounded by MS. I have found that the MS in both of my parents has accentuated the character traits that are the most difficult to manage.

I would desperately like to see Dad living in a house that was better suited to his mobility issues so that he has a better sense of himself and can retain his independence. He's a person who is naturally engaging. People tend to like him and I'd really like to see him socialising with a lot of different people so that he feels like his life has meaning and purpose. But he's been isolating himself a little bit for a while now.

Health-wise I wish I could find something to fix the spasticity issues. Being in a wheel chair is one thing but being unable to get in and out of it or onto a scooter is entirely another problem. His spasticity issues don't allow him to exercise very well either, so together with isolating himself, I feel like all his issues are compounding. He's not adequately addressing his physical health and wellness, let alone his mental health in a particularly holistic way.

At the moment I worry about him every day. I'm not consumed by it, but I certainly mull over the difficulties every day. Both my brother and I live in Sydney and Dad lives about 90 minutes away in Bowral, but it's still too far away for my comfort. I don't think he's confident enough to move away from the base he knows and I understand that. It's only a small town but he knows the lay of the land. I'm happy to work with whatever location he wants to settle in but even then we've got some hurdles to address.

And in the scheme of things he manages himself pretty well. He has set up a daily routine of appointments and activities, so he sort of just plods along. But lately he seems to have hit a bit of a wall... and that's what concerns me the most. He needs people around him supporting him and motivating him and just keeping him generally positive. My brother and I form the framework of Dad's support network and my brother has just had a second baby and I'm very conscious not to load their life up further.

But the other concern is that there's a physical distance between our whole family and we've all got young kids and Dad is missing out on seeing his grandchildren grow up. I know many families weather distance in their relationships but the MS adds a complication to the scenario. Sometimes I feel that the MS has limited his capacity to make decisions and has also massively reduced his confidence. I can't help but feel that the situation would be very different if Dad didn't have MS. And that's heartbreakingly tricky to navigate.

My Dad was an amazing woodworker and sailor and he actually built his own boat when I was younger. My older boy Bruno is taking sailing lessons at his school and is also a keen woodworker and I'd love them to share their passions together. Both Dad and Bruno have quiet and thoughtful personalities and it's these traits that require them to have some continuity in the quality time they spend together so as they can bond, but they haven't had the opportunity to do that yet. It's something I'm campaigning to see happen, especially in having Dad live closer to us, because it would be a great shame if both generations of the family didn't have the opportunity to forge that bond.

Growing up, I remember spending heaps of time together with my own grandparents – and admittedly hating a whole bunch of that time – but it's an important rite of passage and I don't want our kids to miss out. That time spent with your elders is part of the fabric that makes you who you are.

There's no road map for this type of stuff; my brother and I just muddle our way through it, figuring out what works and what doesn't. We get so excited when we devise a brilliant solution – hardly believing that what we've engineered actually works. But similarly, when the wheels fall off with other plans it's fairly demoralising.

And to be honest, we don't want to be making all the decisions for someone else's life either. I speak to my friends about my Dad's current situation and they will say 'just force him to do it.' But Dad isn't old and mad and I couldn't live with myself if I forced him to do something against his will. Dad still has every right to be part of the decision making process. He's still completely compos mentis and capable, so my role has been to become the moderator. We talk things through quite a lot and sometimes I feel like I'm nagging him but it comes out of concern and love and simply wanting a better, more comfortable life for him. Most of the time I'm simply trying to keep him thinking and progressing forward in whatever way we can.

It's one thing to be resigned to living with MS but I never want to see Dad give up. I know that Dad recognises I only have his best interests at heart and I'm very honest and will often admit to him that I feel like I'm nagging him but he knows why I'm doing it. I don't want to see him miserable. I want him to be engaged in life, otherwise what's the point?

It was actually Mum who experienced the greater highs and lows with her disease course. I would see both parents suffer such horrendously bad relapses, where I could never imagine them recovering, but somehow they did. MS will always just stop you in your tracks and keep you wondering.

And the journey of my Mum's diagnosis has been quite different. In the beginning I thought my mum was such an attention seeker! I was back from overseas visiting her and she'd been experiencing a few other health problems and had been constantly sick for at least a year. And even though I had spoken to her regularly, I hadn't actually seen her in some time.

So when I finally returned to Australia for a work trip I was quite alarmed to discover that she'd lost a significant amount of weight. At that point I forced her to go to hospital and she ended up having an emergency hysterectomy. But she woke up from that operation missing the 'vertical hold' on her eye sight. I thought it was certainly very weird but the surgeons kept re-assuring both of us that it was purely because Mum had just endured a major operation. To be honest, I found the surgeons to be quite patronising and unhelpful.

She continued to experience these visual disturbances and some other minor symptoms for a while, despite fully recovering from the earlier surgery. Over twelve months passed and we both went back to our lives but I continued to listen to Mum's range of ailments.

It was 1999 and I was holidaying in New York and pregnant with my first child. Out of the blue my Mum called me to say that she'd just been diagnosed with MS.

All I could say was "Oh fuck. Not you too?" I was bewildered. Dad had been living with MS for about a decade at this point yet I was only just getting my mind around his life when I learned about Mum's diagnosis. The whole situation was unfathomable.

Mum's diagnosis was a lot quicker than Dad's, only taking about a year to be definitive, but I think her symptoms hit her far harder from the start. She was having a lot of problems even walking or talking most days and it sent my brother and I into a panic. We looked at nursing care and full time assisted living but one of mum's bug bears was not having somewhere permanent to live. She'd been free-spirited and travelling all her life but suddenly found herself in a situation where she yearned for a permanent base. And distressingly we quickly found out how limited we were in our options.

It didn't help that Mum wasn't dealing with the diagnosis – let alone the disease – very well. She was like a cut snake at times. She was very sick from her symptoms but she was also very angry.

Mum was the opposite of Dad in that she wanted me to make all the decisions. So I did that for her but I have to admit it all went very badly. It just seemed that every decision I made came back to bite me and for years we were always cranky at each other, making me far less helpful than I could have been. It was a huge lesson for me and from that point on I decided that I never wanted to be the sole person making decisions on my parent's behalf. It had to be a mutually agreeable process.

Like Dad, Mum was around the age of 50 when she was diagnosed and it must be a very difficult age to find out something as life-changing as that. I'm certain that no age is a good age but I just remember Mum and Dad prior to the diagnosis being people who were far calmer and looking forward to winding things back a notch. So to have this spanner thrown in the works would absolutely suck. And I think that's the reason why Mum was so angry. She'd keep telling me how unfair it was because there was too much she had left that she wanted to do in life.

Mum had been an acrobat with Circus Oz and some of my childhood was spent travelling with the circus performers. At the time of her diagnosis she was heavily involved in a multitude of women's performance groups – in fact she still is to this day. She's often invited to teach performance workshops and I think this keeps her going. She doesn't always feel well enough to do it, but I'm so glad that she has such a strong network of support around her and that people always find a way to keep Mum involved in something that feeds her soul.

I can't help but think that Mum allowed herself to get so unwell and run-down prior to her diagnosis and that this contributed significantly to the MS manifesting. Mum was always such a fit and dynamic person and the change I saw in her immediately prior to her operation and the eventual diagnosis of MS shocked me.

Mum tried a few alternative therapies early on but probably the most helpful treatment was focused on diet and exercise. It was a strict routine and the changes were significant. And as soon as some of her symptoms eased she developed a far more positive outlook on life.

Mum's not as fast or agile as she once was but she still confidently gets herself about and has sort of gone back to her free-spirited existence. And while it's good to see her making the most of life, this nomadic existence concerns me greatly. She's been in Adelaide for many years now and has a great network of family and friends to help her and she is hell bent on retaining her independence, but I worry about her long-term strategy.

Mum and Dad haven't really talked much since their divorce nearly 40 years ago, preferring just to get on with their lives independently, but not long ago Mum contacted Dad during one of his low points.

She talked to him about the power of positive thinking; I guess she didn't want to see him dig himself further into a hole with negative thoughts and actions. Her simple message to him was to focus on all the good things in his life. Surprisingly Dad responded to this very well and was grateful for the advice.

Strangely though, Mum wasn't always the one that erred on the side of positivity, but her attitude has really shifted in recent times and it's working for her. It's great to see.

At this point in time I probably worry about Dad more so than Mum. Maybe because Dad has weathered the progression of the disease ten years longer than Mum and he's also ten years older.

Mentally the disease has hit Mum harder because she was always the fitter, healthier person and she couldn't understand why she'd been inflicted with something that curbed her activities in life so rapidly and cruelly. It took her years to get to a point where she could cope better and acknowledge and fight what she had to. Whereas Dad tended to ignore what was going on rather than process what needed to happen – as most men do – and I think the disease took over before he had a decent chance to fight back.

Living with MS hasn't actually changed the fibre of my parents. The MS has made Dad more passive and thinking like a victim of circumstance. I daresay this characteristic has always been there, buried deep down, but being diagnosed with MS seemed to bring it back to the surface for Dad. Mum always did whatever the hell she wanted and she's somehow managed to keep doing that. I often wonder with every new or progressing symptom that affects their lifestyle whether it's just a factor of age or whether it's a symptom of MS? It's not always the easiest thing to differentiate between but I'm getting better at asking myself 'is this aging or is it the MS?'

One of the most difficult things about having both parents with MS is that I've had to distinguish when to be present and there for them or know when to leave them to their own devices. I think kids always have that elastic relationship with their parents but being continually concerned for both parents at once can be very tricky, particularly when they are two very distinct people in their personalities and their outlook on life. And of course, we do all this while trying to manage our own lives and challenges. That's the thing: Life still goes on!

And it continues to be a delicate dynamic to manage because neither parent wants to be a burden and I similarly don't want to be getting in the way of them living their own life. I've learned that I can't take over. I can merely be there to offer support. I remain very vigilant to everything that's going on in their life, but I don't instigate too many changes at all. Again, I'm sure the situation I'm experiencing is no different to anyone with aging parents, but the MS complicates matters a fair deal. Luckily they're both pretty good at taking turns for attention and seem to have a sixth sense about what I can do for each of them at any time.

Lately I've been spending a tremendous amount of time investigating aged care. I'm looking at every avenue, just trying to know every single option out there so as we can make any decisions quickly and depending on the situation at the time. Aged care facilities concern me greatly though. While clinically it might be what Dad needs soon, the atmosphere would swallow him. He's only 73 and has so much spark left in his personality. It's a huge step to take – for everyone – and I don't know what we should do.

I've always thought of a carer as a hands-on role. Someone who assists with the day-to-day management of health and wellness. I wouldn't consider myself a carer but instead a dutiful and sometimes annoying daughter. And I think my support towards my parents is more of an emotional one that I offer. The distance we all live from each other means I can't do the day-to-day tasks that managing a chronic illness requires.

My husband provides the backup I need to support my parents. He's my sounding board and we have many long discussions about their wellbeing. He's absolutely my first port of call and he knows all the players so well. He's been there from the beginning of their disease course.

My brother is also key and we definitely co-share the support. I couldn't imagine not having someone in the same position to talk things over with. And we sort of take turns at providing the support depending on who is feeling emotionally equipped to deal with the various issues that MS brings. To be honest, there have been some times when I've thrown my hands in the air and moaned that I can't look after Mum and Dad any longer and he's stepped up and taken over.

The third key player has been my Dad's best friend. He's been massively supportive and I've been able to go to him to ask advice and share the load. It's been a godsend to bounce ideas off him as he has a relationship with Dad that is different to ours as kids. Having that person who is outside of the family but looking in has been invaluable in providing insight and he often plays devil's advocate. In fact, there's been times when I've felt less crazy or overwhelmed as I've had someone to concur with what I'm seeing or experiencing. Sometimes I wonder if I'm being overprotective and having both my brother and Dad's friend to offer different points of view has kept me grounded. It would be easy to get very stuck in the role we play in the support network – and the same goes for the person actually living with MS – so I find it essential to have a few people you can turn to for different forms of support and advice.

I think I may have been shielded from the initial impact that Dad's diagnosis could have had on me because I was living overseas. But I know my brother felt a real blow. My brother was 15 at the time and I think he felt quite freaked out with what was going on but also maybe a bit responsible. He was a young guy doing what 15 year old boys do and he felt that he created unnecessary stress in Dad's life that then created the MS. We know that it's absolutely not the case but I think he's suffered those thoughts over the years.

Knowing how to look after my parents as they grow older has been tricky. Some days I think I'd happily build a little cottage for Dad out the back but that's a huge step. It's a huge step financially and a huge commitment that would take me from being the dutiful daughter on the sidelines to his permanent carer. And it's not a decision that can be made in isolation either. It effects my husband, my sons, my career and certainly my Dad. But then part of me thinks it's the honourable thing to do, no matter what the consequence.

But if I did it for my Dad I'd absolutely have to do it for my Mum and that's an exceptionally difficult dynamic to manage. We're just not in a position to house them both separately.

Never underestimate the time it takes to look after someone, whether you're being a carer in the traditional sense or the dutiful daughter as I am. Helping Dad, even what little I consider I do, takes up a vast amount of time, so to be honest, the thought of him living with me is a bit daunting. My sons are also at an age where they need a lot of attention and there's always competing pressures. It's nothing overwhelming but life is constantly 'busy.' I feel mean for even saying that Dad's illness puts pressure on me and I certainly feel guilty that we don't think we could manage having Dad live at home. I would dearly love to have him live around the corner, but living under the same roof might be a bit much for everyone concerned.

MS has made me do things that I probably wouldn't have otherwise done. And having not one but both parents with MS has been a huge reminder that life is short. There's things I'm doing now that at a previous time in life I might have considered self-indulgent; but now I see those things as pursuing what is important and mean something to me. How many times do people push aside the things that are really important and instead persist in the things that are expected of them?

MS has also made me less tolerant of people's bullshit. I can't stand the pettiness and selfishness that some people display. When I see the way that people behave so horribly, I can't understand why they'd be that way when I know that everything in life can be so fragile. Life is really short and good health is a blessing.

I'll tell you a secret.... I'm actually quite worried about turning 50. I pretend I don't care but who wouldn't be fearful at turning the same age that both your parents were when they were diagnosed with

MS? And I've got no comparison of how I should be feeling! Of late I've had some problems with my vision. Quite frankly, the problems are most likely what everyone my age experiences, but deep down I worry a bit.

A very small part of me is waiting for that first sign of MS to show up, but then on the other hand I think 'so what?' At the end of the day there's very little I can do about it and whatever happens will happen. I can't expend too much precious energy tying myself in knots over it. I always come back to making the most of what's happening in my life now.

I'm under the impression that there may be a genetic link to MS but it's not necessarily hereditary. My own personal view is that there must be some sort of environmental factor to the onset of MS for both of my parents to be diagnosed. But I can't allow myself to think about the cause of MS too much. I have two beautiful kids, as does my brother, and it's not something you want to spend your life dwelling on. I'm actually quite frustrated that the cause of MS, let alone the cure, is so vague. It just doesn't make sense as a disease.

Funnily enough, when I announced to my mother that I was an ambassador for the Kiss Goodbye to MS campaign she was concerned to think that I might be wearing a lot of red lipstick.

"Emma.... how do we know it's not something in lipstick that causes the disease?" she questioned me. I know it sounds comical and irrational and I don't necessarily agree with her, but at the end of the day her point is that we simply don't know the full cause of MS.

My last set of blood tests came back that I was deficient in vitamin D and that knowledge also provided an irrational sense of dread. Once the doctor explained that really my levels were just comparable to every other person at the end of winter I breathed a sigh of relief. I can't help it though. I'm probably just a little more vigilant than most to the early warning signals of MS.

But I really focus on keeping strong and healthy and trying to look after myself just a little bit better. Again, part of that is being more mature and sensible but for me it's also about not taking life and health for granted. I can't stress enough how counter-productive it is to be paranoid that something bad is going to happen. I've been told that it would certainly be quite acceptable to be paranoid given that both of my parents have MS, but I've decided that living a life full of meaning and sustaining great health and wellbeing is a far more sensible strategy. Putting all that emotional energy into something I can't control is no way to live. There's no point in trying to second-guess what's going to happen next.

I did an interview with a national newspaper last year and it was the first time I'd ever raised with a journalist that both of my parents had MS. I just felt it was the right time to talk about it; MS is such a weird disease and I wanted to bring some awareness to the cause. I've always wanted to leave the world a little bit better than when I entered it…. And maybe this helps.

I don't think I would have discussed my parent's issues publicly if I wasn't finally ready to put some energy into it. I think the more people know about MS, the more people can help. The more stories that are told, the greater the understanding about the effects on life. And with this hopefully comes more research and we can connect more dots to find a cure.

GEOFF KINGSFORD SMITH – FATHER

"We feel everything that our kids feel. When Jillian is down, we're also down. Similarly, when she's happy, we feel happy. It's a feeling that is unique to parents."

Looking back, Jillian's route to diagnosis was actually pretty predictable. In the two years leading up to the diagnosis her life was quite full and chaotic and never shy of drama. She owned a successful digital marketing agency, which she'd established in the height of the GFC, and that kept her incredibly busy. She was attending a lot of business functions and sat on the Board of a local festival. On top of that she was dealing with a fairly messy divorce from her husband, where she had to sell her house and deal with the financial fallout of the marriage split. In the scheme of things, she wasn't any busier or stressed than anyone else, but there was no doubt she was under extreme pressure.

Our other daughter Rachel had decided to travel up to Brisbane for the weekend to visit Jillian. She was about an hour away from arriving when Jillian called her to say she had been admitted to hospital that afternoon and Rachel should just drive directly to the ER. Rachel wasn't overly concerned at the time, thinking that Jillian had just been admitted because of exhaustion or as a precaution.

Once Rachel arrived at the ER, her opinion of Jillian's condition changed rapidly. She became immediately concerned and apparently the whole time Jillian was trying to minimise the severity of situation and re-affirm that nothing was wrong. But it was when, after about an hour of being in the emergency ward with her, that Rachel saw her struggle to get out of bed and walk to the bathroom: Rachel told us later it was that point she started getting really worried. Jillian could barely move her legs and was inching her way along the wall to walk. Her fears were further compounded after watching the various doctors performing the visual and sensation tests.

But it came to a point that evening where there was little else Rachel could do, so she left Jillian in the ward to rest for the night and called us on her way to Jillian's apartment. She urged us to come up to Brisbane the next day as she was staggered by how rapidly Jillian was declining.

It must have been a hard call for Rachel to make because she couldn't really tell us what was going on, what the prognosis might be or really provide any good news. I knew Jillian wasn't dying but in a way, that was more frustrating because we had no information at all to try and work out a solution.

I don't remember multiple sclerosis ever being mentioned. It may have been, but just in passing. On that Friday night when Jillian was admitted to the ER there were so many things that the doctors were considering were wrong with her. It fast became obvious from the details that Rachel was giving me that something quite serious was going on. Jillian had underplayed going to hospital from the start. Clearly even she didn't realise how serious it all was. Rachel was quite concerned and my wife, Vicki, and I made a decision that we should go up to be with the girls the next day. I remember thinking at the time that Jillian was probably just having a 'bit of a turn' and that it wasn't going to be anything too dramatic. We were certainly concerned about her, but never considered that she might have been going through anything that wasn't fixable. I think the worst thing we thought it was going to be was a mini stroke.

We live about five and a half hours from Brisbane and didn't arrive at the hospital until a bit after lunchtime on the Saturday. One of the doctors had only just left from giving Jillian the results of her MRI and she was clearly in a bit of a state. "They think I have MS," she stuttered in shock. I had no idea what MS was. I'd heard of it before – Jillian had grown up participating in the MS Readathons – but I really had no idea what type of condition it was or what it would mean. I really never had much reason to think about it. No one in our family has ever lived with MS. At the time I confused MS with Parkinson's and a few of those other conditions.

Jillian had to be taken off to do more tests but before she left, she thrust a Post-it note with a doctor's number scribbled on it and urged us to call him back to explain what was happening. He eventually came back and told us that Jillian's diagnosis wasn't yet conclusive as they wanted to consult with the neurology department who would most certainly want to do further testing, such as a lumbar puncture and properly read the MRIs. To be honest, he was a bit wishy-washy with what was going on but he gave us little hope that it might be anything else other than MS.

One of the first things Dr Weybil said to us was "It's not a death sentence but it will be a life changer." I believe bad things could happen to anyone and there's always people who are a lot worse off than you are, so at that point I was thinking that whatever MS meant, it was just something we had to face head on and deal with. It was that cut and dry. I was determined to be positive about the situation and encourage the rest of the family to be that way too. The positive people always fair better. If you want to be crook, you'll get crook. But if you want to get better you've just got to take a mind over matter approach. I'm certainly not trying to be naïve in suggesting we could wish the MS away, but I felt that if we could all take a proactive and positive approach, we'd have a far better outcome.

I didn't find out too much about MS until we started Googling and even then I remember being a little bit baffled by all the information. Jillian had been under such an extreme amount of stress in the two years or so leading up to being admitted to hospital, so in my mind I couldn't see it being anything other than a stroke; multiple sclerosis just didn't fit in with our family's medical history.

Jillian had said to me that from the onset the doctor's had thought she may be having a stroke, but I remember weighing things up and thinking that a stroke would be worse in the long run than MS. I'm by no means an expert on strokes but we have some family history with cardio-related ailments and I just felt a stroke would have a far worse impact than MS.

Rachel and I stayed in Brisbane for another two days and Vicki decided to stay on for as long as Jillian needed her. We were three days into this situation and the doctors were still not giving us any information or alternatives. She wasn't even hooked up to a saline drip because they simply didn't know conclusively what was wrong to be able to start a course of treatment.

We really had no reference points to judge what Jillian's outlook might be. The doctors were all talking to us in very extreme terms – which frankly I expected anyway – but regardless, I just didn't know enough about the disease to know what to expect. It dawned on me that I knew two people from my home town that had MS; but I still didn't understand how it affected them. Neither of them were in a wheel chair, so I found it a bit unsettling that Jillian's therapists were talking in these terms.

I would talk to Vicki every night to get updates and I think being away from the constant chaos of the hospital gave me space to think the situation over. While I was concerned about my daughter, I also knew that the MS wasn't life threatening to her. I came to reconcile myself with the cards that she had been cruelly dealt and looked ahead to how we would play those cards. It's the difference between my wife and I, and I daresay most married couples. I was thinking practically and Vicki was thinking emotionally. But Vicki was also immersed in the situation and was constantly trying to work out where to go and what to do next.

We were both dealing with the situation in opposite ways but we were able to play off our strengths and understanding to provide support to each other. I was propping up Vicki with a no-nonsense positive attitude and she was able to download all the information to me every night and vent.

In the lead up to Jillian's diagnosis she would often ring and complain how tired she was. We can now look back on that and understand why, but at the time it was so exasperating. We're all tired and working hard but Jillian would make a fair production out of it. I understand now how much she was underplaying the situation and I daresay she probably still does. Each of us in the family are loathe to even take an aspirin for a headache so we tend to 'suffer in silence.' On the one hand I think it's made us resilient but on the flipside it can also play havoc with getting to the bottom of any serious medical situations.

Taking Control Together:

I remember having to say out loud to someone for the first time "we think Jillian has MS." It's at that point it becomes real. Neither Vicki nor Rachel really knew what to say to other people, primarily because we weren't sure what Jillian wanted people to know. For a while we held the diagnosis back from as many people as possible.

We feel everything that our kids feel. When Jillian is down, we're also down. Similarly, when she's happy, we feel happy. It's a feeling that is unique to parents. We've always felt this way, but Jillian's diagnosis has certainly intensified the feeling. So our life has changed in that we do feel what Jillian is going through. We know how hard it is for her. We want to ensure she's as happy as possible going forward because we do feel her challenges.

This adventure has brought our whole family closer together. Not just our immediate family but also our extended family of relatives.

Jillian's attitude towards many things has changed tremendously since her diagnosis. She's more accepting of things in life and has also created clearer priorities for herself. I'm glad my daughter has changed for the better and found some meaning in what she does now. I remember counselling her one night when she was feeling down that you don't want to worry too much about when things are going bad in your life because it means that things are only going to get better. It's when things are going along TOO well that you want to worry!

One of the hardest things to cope with is seeing a vibrant and ambitious person become increasingly frustrated with their inability to achieve their ongoing goals in life.

We are often frustrated that we can't help more with everyday issues, particularly her cognitive fatigue and seeing how her lack of balance and vertigo is starting to limit some of the activities she can participate in.

The distance that we live from Jillian continues to be a concern for us. We're 600 kilometres away on a large rural property and it's very difficult to just travel anywhere or be there for Jillian at the drop of the hat. Luckily she's fairly independent and has rarely needed us in a hurry. Although I know sometimes she has probably risked her safety to maintain her independence or even refused to tell anyone how bad she was feeling, rather than burden or bother anyone.

We are tremendously grateful for the tight support network that Jillian has built up around her. She has the best group of friends a girl could have and lives in such a tight-knit community, despite the fact that she's residing in one of the biggest cities in Australia. Her friends have been very loyal and supportive; we've made sure they know they can contact us about anything and to be honest, we can breathe easier knowing they are around to protect our daughter.

When I'm in a reflective mood I do get a little sad that things didn't work out differently for Jillian. But as I said before, everyone is dealt different cards in life and you've got to play those cards as you see them. In essence, none of us know what's around the corner. I could see how it might frustrate other parents but I see the changes she's made in her life to prioritise her health and wellbeing and I think this is a far more sustainable path.

VICKI KINGSFORD SMITH – MOTHER

"It can be so hard in those times that Jillian telephones and I can hear the anxiety or distress in her voice. I feel so worried that I'm going to say the wrong thing to her because all I want to do is find some words of wisdom that will make it all better."

I remember walking into Jillian's room that day at the Royal Brisbane and Women's Hospital. She had been placed in the emergency medicine ward overnight, which is really just a holding bay for people until they can work out what's wrong with them. I walked into her room, which already had five other people in beds (all men) and saw Jillian sobbing. Her doctor had only just left from telling her she might have MS and she was clearly in shock and distress.

I backed out of her room because Geoff stepped in immediately and took control of the situation. Jillian tried talking with Geoff and I turned to Rachel to try and work out what was happening. During the six hours it took us to drive up to Brisbane we'd heard nothing at all, so we were playing catch up.

It wasn't until about four days after Jillian's admission to the ER that we started receiving some clarity. This tall and very official looking gentlemen strode up to Jillian's bedside carrying a raft of folders. "I'm Stefan Blum and I'm the neurologist reviewing Jillian's case," explained Dr Blum.

He was pretty precise and clinical, but I guess most medicos are. It wasn't until we started having greater interaction with the physiotherapists, occupational therapists and even one of the younger registrars that we had longer conversations and found out more about Jillian's outlook as far as her mobility and functionality.

Over the years we've had a lot more consultations with Dr Blum and have become grateful for his preciseness and also the fact that every bit of information he gives us is very considered and backed with research. We've often reflected that we'd rather have a doctor tell us how it is than talk in riddles. Having said that we've also become used to the fact that very few doctors or specialists offer up much information unless absolutely required to.

For such a long time we felt disbelief at the entire situation. It took us a bit to process all the probabilities and possibilities of what Jillian's life would be like from that point on. At some stages in consulting with different specialists we were presented with the worst case scenario and we'd go into an immediate panic. But when we had the time to sit down and process everything rationally we figured out that we'd have to take everything day-by-day.

Some of the worst case scenarios we were given were when we had a session with an occupational therapist and she started quizzing me about the set-up of my house. I guess the therapist assumed that Jillian would be going home to live with us on our family farm. We have a newly constructed single story house but it does have two small steps to get from the garage into the house. The therapist counselled us about building ramps and also ensure that our hallways were wide enough for a wheel chair. Even the bathroom taps didn't escape her attention. All her suggestions frightened the hell out of me. We knew Jillian wasn't in great shape but this was quite alarming. We just didn't know enough about MS to know how the disease may affect her life. The therapist was only doing her job and her advice was delivered with empathy, but looking back now we just weren't ready for that sort of information, let alone the change. Thankfully we haven't had to implement ramps or widen hallways either because Jillian has not progressed enough to require a wheelchair.

Jillian spent a bit over three weeks in hospital and the most frightening thing I witnessed was her being unable grip and hold a fork in her left hand and then coordinate it with the knife in her right hand to eat; if she couldn't manage to hold and operate simple objects, how on earth could she manage living by herself? I left the hospital that night in a panic. I couldn't even begin to imagine what we were going to do to manage this disease.

This particular situation was compounded by the fact that we still had very little information on the disease course of MS and because of that we couldn't shape our expectations. Jillian was clearly frightened and she was also becoming increasingly frustrated that her symptoms weren't improving. That evening we jumped up and down and vented our fury to the ward nurses and eventually one of the neurology registrars come in to talk to us. This doctor tried to brush us off as well, but once she realised that she was dealing with two very rational, albeit distraught women, she pulled up a chair and spent some time chatting to us about MS.

One of Jillian's biggest concerns was when she might be able to be released from hospital so she could get back to attending to her clients and running her business. Whether right or wrong, the registrar quickly put the brakes on that activity. She counselled Jillian that it would likely be quite a number or weeks, or even months, before she'd be able to return to any type of work. I think it was finally the first time that someone had started managing our expectations. It's one thing to be positive but we also needed to be realists.

We were also advised that MS was just such a difficult disease to predict the nature of. Everything would constantly be in a state of flux. The fact that she couldn't walk at that point or use her hands properly may well change the next week. And in fact it did. She still has some mobility issues and finds gripping with her left hand a little more challenging, but no one would ever realise this and she manages wonderfully by herself most of the time.

Other than all the drama that was going on with the diagnosis of MS, Jillian was also in a very undesirable situation at the hospital itself. For some time, she was in the Emergency Medicine ward, which is full of men and women with a variety of illnesses. It was complete chaos and to be honest a bit eye-opening. She couldn't get the rest or specialised neurological care she needed. She was terribly upset at the diagnosis and had to contend with a ward full of men staring at her all day. It wasn't until about ten days later that they finally found her an all-female room and even that was short-lived.

I felt like we were waging two wars. One against the diagnosis of MS and one against the public hospital system.

In those first few weeks I seemed to live in a state of complete shock. The day the physiotherapist wheeled a variety of walking aids to her bedside and taught her how to use each of them was an eye-opener. She couldn't walk further than about ten metres but on the bright side she had a array of implements to choose from to support her!

Nothing prepares you to witness someone teaching your child how to use a mobility aid. I'm not talking about crutches and a broken leg, I'm talking about walkers and wheelchairs. For a mother to watch her daughter – who is 20 years younger – struggle with something many of us take for granted is absolutely heartbreaking. And her mobility issues where changing from one week to the next and that was quite frightening. We had no answers and no solutions.

During those weeks in hospital we came to find a nice routine of going downstairs to the coffee shop each morning after doctor's rounds. It was our escape; our time where we could both talk quietly and try to cling to a bit off sanity away from the wards.

Hospitals are all about 'worst case scenarios.' The doctors and specialists have a duty (and surely a protective imperative) to explain the worst thing that could happen. But on the flip side, we've come to understand a little more about MS and that everyone's symptoms are different and changeable, as are their attitudes and expectations.

The fear of the unknown is a huge and scary situation to manage and the diagnosis can be a very lonely place for everyone concerned. Certainly the patient with the condition can feel isolated but I also felt very alone. For those first few weeks in hospital, Jillian didn't want the world knowing what was wrong. I think she was still trying to process the information herself. She also didn't want people feeling sorry for her or thinking she was less capable. So I only spoke to Geoff and Rachel about what was going on. It wasn't until Jillian's third week in hospital that my sister-in-law called. She was interstate visiting with her own daughter, an occupational therapist.

"Simone wants to talk to you," Judy said as soon as she got on the phone. Judy passed the phone over to Simone, who immediately said "Vicki, I don't know how to ask this so I'm just going to come out with it. Does Jillian have MS?"

I was stunned and all I could answer with was "how do you know?" Up until that point we'd only ever said that Jillian was in hospital having scans and awaiting results.

"I work in the field and everything just added up," stated Simone.

I confirmed the diagnosis to Simone and as heartbreaking as it was to say out loud it was also a relief. I could finally talk to someone else about it. I hadn't realised how desperately I needed to confide in someone else.

From that point on though, I know I've adopted a different persona when I talk about Jillian's MS. I become very clinical about it all. That's certainly the way Jillian talks about it too, so I'm unsure whether I'm following her lead or we're all just protecting ourselves a little from the emotion of the situation. I don't know if it's the healthiest approach to take, but for better or worse it's worked for us. I have developed a series of standard and rehearsed responses to most questions. When people (outside of our close family and friends) enquire about Jillian I know they're mostly being polite in asking. They don't really have a vested interest and the information doesn't really effect their own lives anyway. I've come to learn that about people; if it doesn't impact their own lives then they really don't care about what you have to say or how you're feeling. Everything is just polite conversation.

I'm really just a carer-from-afar. And it's such a difficult role to play. I'd much rather be there supporting Jillian in person but the simple fact is that we have both happily chosen to live 600 kilometres apart. It can be so hard in those times that Jillian telephones and I can hear the anxiety or distress in her voice. I immediately jump to thinking the worst possible thing has happened until she explains she's just having a bad day. I feel so worried that I'm going to say the wrong thing to her because all I want to do is find some words of wisdom that will make it all better. But those words rarely exist.

We all feel the same. Sometimes we really struggle with finding the right things to say. But I also know that Jillian realises that there's no magical solution and isn't looking for us to provide it. She generally just wants to vent and get whatever is worrying her off her chest; she just wants to be heard.

To be honest, I don't think this dynamic will change much over time. I don't think experience will teach us anything because every experience and situation is going to be different and it's just in our nature to want to 'fix things.'

However, when it comes to how Jillian cares for herself or is choosing a treatment plan, we try to encourage her to discuss it with us. We've taken the path that it's her body and her choice but we still want to be there to discuss options and provide an opinion. I don't feel at all conflicted giving my opinion when it comes to these things as I know Jillian researches everything and is good at seeking medical opinions. We would never be offended if she didn't take the advice. But I also think it's easier to provide advice about concrete and tangible issues such as medications or procedures. It's the emotional stuff that is harder.

We've certainly reprioritised many things in our life. Things that we may have considered quite important only a few years ago are really quite insignificant now. What we devote our time to is a great example of this. We've stopped being 'too busy' to do the things we enjoy or 'too busy' to look after our own health. And with this reprioritisation has come a change in our value system. Friendships mean more to us than they ever have and I think we are just generally more empathetic to other people's problems than we used to be; we understand now what they might be going through.

Interestingly, we're also more discerning as to the charities we support now. We make more informed decisions when donating and our preference is to support causes that further research.

I know a lot of our friends and family don't fully understand what we're going through or how we cope mentally and emotionally with everything, but Geoff, myself and the girls are constantly reminding ourselves that there are many worse off than us. I think it's become an unofficial family motto!

I've talked to a few other parents who have kids with MS but I didn't necessarily find it helpful. Just as MS is different for everyone, so too are our attitudes to coping with it. The mere fact that you share a child with MS doesn't make a meeting of the minds and doesn't mean that you'll both share the answers to the situation.

The hardest thing I've found is that feeling you can't talk to anyone about what's going on. Everyone in this day and age have their own problems to deal with, so why would they be concerned about someone else's issues? And frankly, why would I want to add to the load?

This situation with Jillian has certainly made us think about our own health and how we and she is going to cope down the track. You can't quite describe to someone how to value what they do have when they are healthy.

The whole thing has brought us back down to earth and forced us to examine our values and the way we live. Living a simple life without too much stress is important now.

We're now much more aware of the frailty of life. We've experienced how easily something we take for granted can be taken away. It's also put our own life into perspective in many ways.

Our family has gone through some heartbreaking family deaths over the years that by all accounts forced us make some changes, but Jillian's diagnosis was more defining. Death makes you change some things about life and its permanence is horrendous. But things do go on. I think when you're caring for someone close to you with a chronic illness, the impact is constant. You can see the daily effects and struggles. And particularly when it's your own daughter – your own flesh and blood – you see and feel what's happening daily.

We do worry about Jillian's future as we are all getting older. Most parents would raise their children to the best of their abilities, knowing (or perhaps hoping) that at some point in life their kids can then step up and look after them in their old age. A reversal of the family dynamic, so to speak.

But with Jillian's diagnosis we've had to re-assess certain financial plans in our own business because we don't want Jillian to weather any additional burden. She never expected us to continue looking after her as an adult; in fact we've had many a joke about how if we didn't watch ourselves she wouldn't fulfil her duties as a good daughter and look after us in our old age! But things haven't quite worked that way and re-engineering a succession plan and financial strategy is something we want to do to protect both of our kids.

Jillian has completely changed her lifestyle to deal with both the MS and the breast cancer she was diagnosed with ten weeks later. She exercises daily, she eats an MS approved diet and she gets the rest she needs. I feel she is a living model for a healthy lifestyle. She has changed the way we think.

We are extremely proud of Jillian and the way she has faced life since the diagnosis of both diseases – impossibly close together. Jillian, like most people living with MS hasn't given up but has instead carried on with her life as normally as possible. She rarely complains but we know she suffers greatly at times and is clearly frustrated by how the disease has limited her life in some ways. But we feel it's important that she keeps her head high and tries to lead a fulfilling and 'normal' life and it's the special network of friends she has surrounding her that bolster her in doing this. We are most grateful to those people for what they continue to do for our daughter, especially given that we can't be there in person all the time.

Dear Mum and Dad

Being my parents must be the hardest job in the world and you do it with such ease. The process of being diagnosed with MS was such a whirlwind one; I never had a chance to think about what was happening. Back then I seriously just put one foot in front of the other. But I'll never forget that hideous day three years ago when I'd gone in to have an investigative mammogram. It was only ten weeks after being told I had MS and the doctors didn't beat around the bush in telling me I also had breast cancer. I sat alone in the cab going home. All I could think was how the heck am I going to tell you? This will destroy you.

But it didn't. It took me a few hours to pull myself together enough to dial your number but you both had a quick 'oh shit' moment and then rallied around me. I can only imagine the anguish you felt that night, 600 kilometres from me in Brisbane and wondering what the future would hold.

Over the last three years it has been your strength and courage and humour and support that has kept me from coming unhinged. There's not a day that goes by that I'm not tremendously grateful for the way you have raised me and the resilience you have instilled. But I do it all for you. This book is for you. The fact that I keep putting one foot in front of the other – even on the shitty days – is for you, and I couldn't imagine any better way to honour everything you've done for me.

Making you proud of everything I do is the force that drives me. Whenever I have a decision to make, my guiding principle is 'will it make my family proud?' Early into my MS diagnosis I set my sights on becoming an advocate for awareness of this ridiculous disease. It's not the sexiest, nor easiet role, and I'll certainly never become a millionaire from it, but it has enriched my life beyond words. And I couldn't do this without your support and backing. You inspire me to push forward and you cheer me in everything I do.

I know all this support comes at a cost to you. And I know I still stress you terribly. But we've had this conversation before and I'll say it quite publicly again: I wouldn't change a thing in my life. MS is a shitty disease but it's made me a better person. I can recognise and be grateful for the good times and extraordinary things. I can cut through all the garbage to see the real priorities in life. And I've learned not to waste a second. Everything counts now.

And I hope the positive change in me has also inspired you to re-adjust your own perceptions as to how a life well lived should play out. I see it in you even if you don't fully recognise it yourself. We were always a close family but now more so than ever. And that's the best feeling in the world.

Thank you for always believing in my dreams. I love you Mum and Dad.

Jillian xx

PAUL MURNANE - HUSBAND

"I've spent most of my life professionally solving problems and this is one problem I can't solve. And when you attempt to solve it, you're inclined to think that you're doing it entirely alone."

Over the past 35 years, Paul Murnane has forged a notable career as a corporate advisor and company director. He has been a director of Citibank and Goldman Sachs and was a partner at Russell Reynolds Associates, a leading global executive leadership and search firm. He is the current Chairman of MS Research Australia.

In addition to this, Paul is a company director or advisor for a variety of for-profit and not-for-profit organisations. He's long been interested in overseas poverty alleviation in developing countries and sits on two boards whose focus is to address these issues. He co-founded the Australian Scholarships Foundation to boost the efficiency and effectiveness of Australia's not for profit organisations. On the other end of the spectrum he's heavily involved in organisations that develop music, sitting on the board of the Australian String Quartet and also the well-known think tank The Sydney Institute.

Paul's lengthy personal experience with MS – after the diagnosis of his wife Annie nearly 20 years ago – has made him only too aware of the realities of MS. He now uses this knowledge to drive his passion and determination to secure

successful MS research outcomes for Australians with MS.

***

Iwas meeting with John Studdy on the day that Annie got 'THE' phone call. John was a luminary in his field and sat as chairman of some of the most stellar corporates in the country but that day I was meeting with him in my offices about a business matter. I knew Annie was seeing the neurologist for the results of her MRI and I'd asked her to call me as soon as she knew anything. Neither of us were terribly worried and our attitude was that we'd simply deal with whatever the prognosis was. To be honest we'd just gone through the process of ruling out that it was a brain tumour or something similarly as sinister, so frankly MS was probably going to be a relief.

During my meeting with John, Annie called and confirmed that she had MS. I don't remember her being upset; in fact she mentioned she was going out to do something else and she'd see me at home later and we could talk about everything then. I wasn't stunned, I wasn't upset but I was concerned and it must have been written on my face. John merely asked "Bad news?"

I turned to John and said "Annie's just been diagnosed with MS."

"I happen to be the Chairman of the National Multiple Sclerosis Society of Australia," announced John. "So excuse me for just a moment and we'll sort this out."

With that he grabbed my phone and made a call. Within about ten minutes this bloke arrived at the foyer of my offices, sweating and panting. I came to find out it was the CEO of the MS Society of NSW and he'd run from their offices a few blocks away to hand deliver an information pack. And from that moment on I've been involved in a journey with MS, not only with my wife, but on an organisational level as well.

***

Annie, like me, has had a couple of careers throughout her life. When I first met her in our late twenties she was working with the CEO of Brambles Industries but my roles in investment banking meant we travelled and moved around a lot.

When I met Annie there was no evidence at all of MS. She hadn't experienced any symptoms since her early twenties but we now look back and realise she's probably had MS since her teen years. It wasn't until her late 40s that she was diagnosed.

Growing up, Annie spent a lot of time on a sheep property in Australia's Riverina area. She remembers that she was always more affected by the heat out there than her older sister was. Another thing she remembers is that as a keen competitive tennis player she became increasingly frustrated when she noticed that she was missing the occasional tennis ball despite it landing right in front of her; lack of proprioception and the onset of some visual issues are a classic sign of MS. But at that age, you're not sure what's normal and what isn't, so Annie didn't bother mentioning it to anyone, let alone get it checked out. She thought all kids had problems like that. And frankly back when Annie was a teenager the medical profession wouldn't have been able to easily diagnose MS anyway.

She recounted a story to me about how she was backpacking through Europe in her early twenties with a friend and she started to experience problems with her vision. Apparently everything just suddenly turned black and white and soon after she completely lost her eyesight in one eye. Her father organised for her to see a doctor on Harley Street but by the time she was able to meet the specialist, the symptom had vanished. Incidentally, the doctor put it all down to her being a homesick kid and slid her a bottle of Valium across his desk. At this Annie stood up, looked at him indignantly and casually dropped the bottle into his waste basket as she exited with instructions not to bother sending an account for his services as she wouldn't be paying for his lack of advice!

We can reflect on the stories now and see that all these issues were the start of relapsing remitting MS.

Jumping forward to 1977: I was working in New York, we were living in Connecticut and pregnant with our first child when Annie started walking with a limp and feeling just a bit 'off' in general.

She said her eyes weren't working properly and her writing had become jerky but she put it down to being some seven months pregnant. We had made an appointment at a clinic close to where we lived, just to check everything out. Quite coincidentally, the doctor we were to consult with pulled up at the same time as we did and watched Annie walk across the carpark. At that moment, he didn't realise that he was watching his next patient trying to walk, but he watched her knowing something wasn't right. In fact, we didn't find out this little anecdote until some time later when he included the incident in his report back to another set of specialists; he was certain there was a neurological issue unfolding.

But even then, Annie still went undiagnosed. Back in the 70s, there was only an experimental MRI machine in New York City. I was fortunate enough through my role at Citibank to have access to the best specialists in the country and the most esteemed medical facilities, yet no one was able to pinpoint what was wrong with Annie. The official comment – and remember we're going back forty years – was that Annie was experiencing a 'happening.' They couldn't prove one way or the other what was wrong. I'm unsure why a lumbar puncture wasn't performed as it may have shed a bit more light on things.

Not long after this our first daughter was born and eventually we moved back to Australia. Our second daughter followed not too many years later and Annie decided to pursue a career in IT (as well as French language studies at University) given that we were a bit more settled in Australia. We still travelled extensively for my work, and Annie's studies were quite rigorous too, but generally speaking, her previous symptoms were stable.

It wasn't until the mid 90's – when she was much more established in her career – that the symptoms flared again. Her eyesight started to play up again, this time bringing double vision and fatigue. Annie was convinced it was from spending long hours in front of computers and her own optometrist joked that at her age it was about time she started wearing glasses!

So she was prescribed a pair of spectacles and again, in true Annie style she marched back to the optometrist six weeks later to tell her how useless they were. The problem persisted so her GP then referred her to a specialist optician who had coincidentally, or maybe luckily, spent six years working in an MS clinic in London.

She listened to Annie and took one look at her eyes.

"I want you to see a neurologist immediately," explained this doctor. "I think you have MS."

Every time we saw a specialist overseas for the symptoms Annie was experiencing we would ask if it could possibly be MS. Even years later, one of Annie's earlier Australian GPs told me that he had toyed with the idea that what she was facing might be MS. Still no one took her symptoms further; I believe there just wasn't the awareness around the disease or diagnostic capabilities to do much more than speculate. I've since learned that many other people at the time had very similar difficulties in getting diagnosed. Many weren't taken seriously and by the time they were able to see a specialist the symptoms were no longer presenting themselves so the doctors had nothing to look at.

Annie has always been a person who looked at the glass as being half full, so she really just got on with life throughout all of this. We finally obtained a conclusive MRI diagnosis in 1996 from a neurologist in Sydney, who is still her neurologist to this day.

***

There was definitely a sense of relief at knowing what it was. Firstly because we finally had a name for what Annie was experiencing. Secondly, she felt vindicated at what she'd been feeling. She knew that her symptoms were real; and finally, we both knew that MS wasn't terminal so we knew we could figure out how to manage it all.

At that stage she was still quite capable and working full-time. The kids were also old enough to understand what was going on and manage themselves. And because her symptoms were primarily relapsing and remitting episodes, we didn't really notice any immediate impact on our life.

Even though Annie had been diagnosed in Australia, she'd had a decade of access to the MS societies in America while she was trying to work out for herself what was wrong. Some twenty years ago she found the information she could secure from the States far more detailed and helpful than what was then available in Australia. And remember, this was in the time before we could jump straight onto the internet to search for information. Annie would spend hours talking to specialists and organisations in America to get the information she needed.

The children were largely aware of what MS was and understood the disease was predominantly a condition that effected females. We had some discussions about whether MS was genetic or hereditary in nature not long after Annie was diagnosed but we've really never talked about it much since. We just got on with living life. The kids were such a terrific help though. There was never a fuss; they just pitched in, everything got done and I think we all tried to keep our lives looking much as they had prior to the diagnosis. It was that routine in fact, that if one of the girls was helping Annie with an injection it might literally done on the fly during television commercials or as they were racing out the door to go somewhere. We're just not the type of family to make a big deal out of things.

We certainly immersed ourselves in the disease from an educational level so we could work out what our options were but my own involvement in the various MS organisations was as about as serendipitous as the other events throughout my career; if it hadn't been John Studdy sitting in front of me the day Annie was diagnosed, I may never have had anything other than a loose association with MS Australia.

But John did telephone me about six months after that fateful day and asked if I'd be willing to sit on the board of the Multiple Sclerosis Society of NSW. I reluctantly agreed and for the next nine years I threw myself in the services side of the organisation, learning a tremendous amount about how everything operated. Subsequently

I became Chairman.

I'm a strategic thinker and one day I set about plotting on a map all the branches of the state MS Societies that were adjacent to the Murray River in both New South Wales and Victoria. In some instances only a few kilometres separated the branches, yet they were operated as separate entities and could offer different services. It was completely nuts and I remember showing the map to our Board. Everyone realised there were two distinct state operations adjacent to each other and doubling up on resources.

That map was the start of a big journey for me. I could see so many opportunities to reallocate resources for greater efficiency and impact. We didn't need two different accounting departments, two different HR departments and so on. If we could re-engineer the way we operated the adjacent state MS Societies we could redistribute those resources to the front line to help people with MS fight the disease.

I subsequently became the inaugural chairman of Multiple Sclerosis Limited, which was formed when we merged the Victorian, NSW and ACT Societies. I pushed for the amalgamation because to me it made better sense for one larger organisation to offer more services to more people in more places, hopefully avoiding duplication of resources.

The other area I was stunned about from my early days in the MS movement and that fundamentally fuelled my drive for change was the fragmented approach to MS research. Multiple sclerosis was just a poor cousin compared to other diseases; there was no strong national commitment to finding research funds for treatments or a cure. Yet the MS Societies had a proud history of funding MS research dating back to 1963.

Undoubtedly MS became more relevant to me because of Annie's diagnosis. I realised any of the research gains we made at that time would help future generations but the further I delved into the worlds of disability, medical research and aged care I formed the opinion that it was misleading for organisations to lay claim to the exercise of finding cures through research when clearly the bulk of the money necessarily went into services, often accessible only to a small group of people living with that disease. On top of that, I could see the services were mostly confined to people living in metro areas, leaving rural families (about 40% of the total) without support.

Maybe because of my background as an investment banker I focussed on how services and research were funded. There was money for services and there was money for research and sometimes those two streams came from the same donor but ended up in different pots. Obviously commitment to research takes a long time for any dividend to be paid and it invariably takes really big bucks to make any difference. With services, the need is more immediate and tangible and therefore an easier, more understandable 'pot' for the Societies to direct their funding into. And while I rationally understood the reasoning behind all of that, I couldn't help but consider it wrong. There was no long term game plan for increasing fundraising efforts into research.

I remember writing an email to our board in 2002 and declaring that while I wasn't a medical researcher and had even less idea how to set up a research institute, I believed the fundraising efforts towards MS research were tokenism at best unless we began to think strategically and big. I went on to say "if we could wave our magic wands would we simply be fiddling around the fringes of MS research in the way that we are today?"

I vowed to set up an organisation dedicated to MS research from that moment. I had a whole series of ideas (admittedly some of them quite whacky) on how we could establish the organisation. Unbeknownst to me, a small group of people from several other MS Societies were thinking along the same lines but hadn't yet taken it to the national level.

One thing led to another and I eventually spoke with the head of The Garvan Institute, whom I knew quite well.

"I think you should come have a cup of coffee with me," he suggested when I told him I wanted to start a research foundation.

"I'd really like to change your mind on this one. You have no idea what you're getting yourself into!" He was only joking but I knew we were embarking on an enormous task.

We all pushed forward and on the same weekend of the Bali Bombings in October 2002, a group of us met in Bondi and agreed to form an independent national research body. Over the next eighteen months considerable work led to the establishment of MS Research Australia, with Simon McKeon, an ex-board member of MS Victoria, as its inaugural chairman and Jeremy Wright as its CEO.

***

Historically much medical research has been siloed and researchers would study the discipline they were expert in, without much cross-talk between disciplines and institutions. This approach was common for all medical research, not just MS research.

Despite these limitations, much important work was undertaken before 2004. Australia has always been home to world-class experts in many areas of MS research, including immunology, genetics, neurobiology and integrated medicine.

Previously, the competitive research funding model made collaboration more difficult, and some duplication of research efforts inevitably existed. Nationally coordinated MS research networks and collaborations were more difficult to establish, affecting the number of high-quality collaborative outcomes. The complex nature of MS makes cross-disciplinary collaborations especially important for bringing diverse expertise to a project.

Before 2004, MS research lacked a common national direction and received relatively little funding. MS Research Australia was to change this.

In 2004 the existing National MS Research Foundation was converted into MS Research Australia, with changed goals, roles and governance. The first strategic objectives were to develop major sponsorship funding campaigns, whilst also establishing the governance structures and a portfolio of research themes. MS Research Australia wanted to substantially increase available funding and realign the MS research effort. This would require a focused MS research funding campaign and a revised research structure.

By 2006 the research investment had nearly doubled to more than $1 million – the highest allocation MS researchers had seen in ten years. The public profile had risen and an active Board of Directors had been established. Several important partnerships had been initiated that would come to make a vital contribution to supporting MS research, including Macquarie Bank Foundation, the Trish MS Research Foundation and the grassroots fundraising body Foundation 5 Million.

The founding objectives of the organisation required a new approach to MS research – a challenge that produced an innovative solution.

MS Research Australia and the researchers would establish a network of national research platforms, clinicians, and other specialists and researchers from around the country who all worked together. In this way, research infrastructure and data could be shared. Granting schemes would encourage collaboration and focus on large scale programmes and projects that were comprised of multidisciplinary teams.

MS Research Australia would provide research strategies and direction, funding, governance and communication. The immediate research questions focused on the genetics of MS, the blood-brain barrier, and repair and regeneration.

The approach was to contribute to MS on a worldwide scale, build on Australian strengths and importantly, provide benefits to people with MS by making research breakthroughs. Australia would be actively searching for a cause, aggressively identify new treatments, and addressing the symptoms of MS. Scientists would see a much higher level of commitment to MS research, new opportunities to collaborate and exchange ideas and more stable funding.

In just ten years, MS Research Australia has grown from a small organisation to an important and well-respected national funder and facilitator of MS research in Australia. Grants have been awarded across Australia and New Zealand and platform projects incorporate researchers from both Australia and New Zealand, providing support for the best MS researchers within all the major universities, institutes and hospitals.

Since 2004 MS Research Australia has funded more than $22 million in Australian research endeavours. About 29% of this funding was sourced from the MS Societies, with the balance coming from MS Research Australia's independent fundraising efforts. This includes more than 150 separate investigator-led research grants in all states and territories, totalling more than $14 million overall, with an additional $8 million allocated to directed collaborative research projects known as platforms.

Importantly this nationwide growth in funding support is also reflected in the Australian research output for the same period. Both the quality and quantity of research produced by Australian academics has grown enormously, both from MS Research Australia support and through other funding resources.

***

I was pretty confident that the organisation would grow rapidly once we turned our focus purely to the area of research and didn't divert our attention into the services side of the equation, which the State branches were still managing. And with our undivided attention, we were able to take the available funding for research from $440,000 in 2004 right up to more than $3 million in 2013.

As the research arm of MS Australia, the peak federation representing Australians with MS, MS Research Australia's activities are truly national. Our segregation from the state MS Societies from the beginning allowed it to focus nationally and really deliver outcomes that the whole country could benefit from.

While all this was going on, Annie's own disease course was progressing and about ten years after her diagnosis she decided to retire from work altogether. It was mainly her eyesight that was limiting her and she would also experience a little bit of short term memory loss.

And in fact, for many years after her retirement she would still do things like ice skating and dancing, but there came a time when her eyesight would play havoc with her balance. Without balance, ice skating and dancing and those sort of things aren't much fun.

She only stopped driving about four years ago and it was certainly something she elected to give up for safety reasons. Shortly after that, her mobility decreased further but it wasn't actually a specific symptom of MS that was limiting her mobility; she'd had a few nasty falls and the ensuing operations on her knee put her first into a walking frame and later a wheel chair. So within a three year period she'd gone from being independent to always needing assistance because of her severe lack of stability after the knee injuries. We decided to get some help for Annie each day because it was just too risky having her be by herself all day. She'd already sustained so much through three different knee surgeries and the rehabilitation and her memory was also a bit off at times, so the family felt much more re-assured having someone at home with her. Most days I'd drop her at a friend's place or a great day care facility on my way to work and other days she'd have a carer stay with her at our home.

Then a year ago Annie had a stroke whilst she was sleeping. She was immediately hospitalised for this and unfortunately hasn't been home since. She's transitioned between neurology wards and the rehabilitation hospital and following her assessment as high care, we've recently just found a nursing home that can provide her the permanent care she now needs.

She still has significant cognition issues but to be honest, it's hard to discern what has been caused by the stroke and what is actually the MS progressing. There's no remaining visible stroke symptoms other than paralysis in her right arm and leg, which she hadn't had any issues with prior to the stroke. She has good days and bad days cognitively. Some days she'll be asking me to help her pack for a trip we'd planned twenty years ago and other days she's speaking fluent French to her physio.

When I look back on Annie's disease course I think we've been very fortunate. Her MS course has largely been benign. As my career evolved, Annie, the kids and I were able to travel widely as a family and due to my senior roles I've also been fortunate to have considerable autonomy so as I could help Annie with anything she needed. Over the years she's had very few relapses that were dramatic enough for her to be rushed to hospital. Most of the time we could manage them from home and although we'll never know, I'm hopeful that the treatments she was taking and continues to take for MS were beneficial in warding off any significant progression.

The stroke was caused by atrial fibrillation, a type of heart rhythm disorder called an 'arrhythmia.' Atrial fibrillation – or AF – is a condition that occurs when there is a fault in the electric activity in the heart muscle, causing the heart to beat irregularly and in an uncoordinated way. Our cardiologist explained that many people have AF but often the first time they know about it is when they have a stroke and die. We were at least able to catch Annie's and work with it as quickly as possible.

Annie's own attitude towards chronic illness was also her biggest asset. From day one of Annie's journey with MS she just put her head down and got on with things. This is not to deny she didn't have her "down" days due to frustrations with her MS. No one ever knows how they're going to react to a life changing diagnosis but Annie was my hero; she was just so resilient.

I remember us discussing the topic of resilience one day. She wondered if living with a chronic illness made a person more resilient or if people were perhaps pre-programmed to be disposed with resilience? I think it's a really interesting topic and something I've studied professionally for a long time. The short answer is we don't know. Clearly you have to adjust and change to accommodate the new circumstances but some people don't make that adjustment as well as others. I've seen plenty of cases where the person living with MS becomes very dependent on other people but on the flip side I've seen MS make people stronger and more courageous.

I'm not a scientist but I've had access to a lot of bright and dedicated ones in the field and over the years I've become relatively well-versed in MS research. I'm really encouraged to think that in the next decade remitting relapsing MS (RRMS) will be extremely well controlled by drug therapies. We've already got about a dozen treatments available for RRMS with new drugs offering fewer side effects being released each year. And the great benefit of controlling or at least significantly slowing RRMS is that it then slows down the onset of progressive forms of MS. And by slowing the progressive forms we will see over time the ripple effect of less demand on the services that the MS societies offer as well as a decreased need for government spending across those services. My hope is we can instead funnel these savings into researching progressive forms of MS, in many ways the 'final frontier' of MS research.

For the first time in my twenty years of dealing with MS we're finally seeing the attack on progressive forms of MS, similar to the attack we saw on relapsing-remitting MS two decades ago. Until recently, it was one area that the researchers found very difficult to tackle. But now, scientists and drug companies are finally seriously contemplating what causes the progress of MS and how to develop treatments. My expectations are that we'll have major advances in progressive MS once the focus is reset.

There's a lot more emphasis now on translating research, including social and applied research, into clinical treatments. Previously much of the research centred around lab work on genetics and the like, and while still important, it's encouraging to see clinicians pairing with the researchers to collaborate on projects. It's happening all around the world and it's a big breakthrough for people living with MS.

You see it happening at hospitals now. It's increasingly likely your neurologist is part of a research team. We see it done particularly well at places like the Garvan Institute and the Millenium Institute where the clinicians and the scientists are working right beside each other. You walk into a scientist's lab and in the room next door a clinician might be seeing a patient. It's a very promising sign as to the progression of MS research.

On the other hand, government research grants are being reduced drastically. Only 14% of all National Health and Medical Research Centre (NHMRC) grant applications were approved in 2014. Basically more than 80% of researchers who applied for a federal government grant were unsuccessful. And this will be a big problem for our country.

MS Research Australia intends to be heavily involved in the Medical Research Future Fund debate. In 2015, the Australian Government proposed to establish a $20 billion Medical Research Future Fund to provide secure funding for medical research over the coming decades. It will facilitate Australia maintaining a world class medical research sector, with access to cutting edge innovation and clinical breakthroughs in our hospitals, and would be the largest fund of its type in the world.

Our board is very passionate about making governments understand that we need to turn things around in medical research; that every dollar spent now curing diseases will potentially reduce the cost of treating or maintaining hospitals and medical care in the future.

I think MS Research Australia has been phenomenally successful in its first decade of operations. We've been witness to so many exciting breakthroughs, not just in Australia but globally. It's now considered the largest non-government funder of MS research in the country, which is a huge leap from the paltry $400,000 we were able to funnel into projects ten years ago.

What's really pleasing is that it's only one of twelve not-for-profit research foundations that can award the very prestigious Category One funding. And this Category One status is really important because those funds generally seed additional funding from other sources. It's as if we've given a project our 'tick of approval,' so to speak, and other funders such as universities and hospitals feel confident in investing further. In basic terms, a project supported by MS Research Australia generally goes on to get at least three times the monetary support we provide. For some interesting and cutting edge projects, that could jump up to 27 times the funding, partly because of the research governance approach we have applied and the projects we support. The work of MS Research Australia has definitely changed the landscape of medical research and particularly the perception of MS in Australia.

***

I think the carer's role can be tough and certainly exploited by governments. Most people in that support role don't get paid for the work they do, yet it's a responsibility that is a complete necessity for many. I think it would be fascinating, if one day, everyone in that carer role turned around and said to the hospitals and the governments, "here you are - you look after this person." Just for 24 hours I'd love to see what would happen if all the carers in Australia walked away. It would be a shambles and would have a diabolical effect on the health and welfare system.

Institutionalising people isn't the solution. In my mind the solution lies in creating a system with flexibility, and by its very nature this will be quite complex. The assistance currently offered for home care help, for example, just isn't enough. It's token at best and I can understand why many people are forced to retire from work so as they can attend to a family member who needs further care. But who can afford to do that?

The most practical piece of advice I ever received was to seek out the best doctors and medical advice that you can find. Never hesitate to shop around to find the specialist that resonates with you and your lifestyle. And above all, be very demanding. You're placing your, or your loved one's health in their hands, so you're allowed to be demanding.

And then once you've done all that, ensure the medical team are communicating amongst each other. The neurologists, GPs, pharmacists, physios, opticians, surgeons – and the list goes on – need to be talking to each other about correlating the treatment plan.

Annie and I formed a club called the OPP Club, which stands for

'Other People's Problems.' We found there were a lot of people who just didn't understand MS and were very negative about living with it. We decided from the onset of Annie's diagnosis that it was in fact the other people who had the problem, not Annie or me! We tend to ignore people who create issues now; people who offer 'free advice' in the form of outlandish suggestions or treatment ideas. "It's all in your mind" and "Your balance would be fine if you stopped drinking" are two memorable (and ignorant) comments!

And most importantly I've learned you can never lose your sense of humour. You'd probably never ever get out of bed again if you lost your sense of humour when dealing with MS.

I remember trying to explain to a colleague what it was like living with someone who has MS. I recounted how that very morning I had woken up early and it was still dark but I could feel Annie moving in bed. I asked quietly if she was awake.

"Yes," she replied tentatively. "I'm just seeing what's working today." She was gently moving each part of her body, seeing how it reacted, what her brain was telling the various limbs to do and what the sensations were. To actually wake up every morning and have to wonder about what the day was going to be like and what you might or might not be able to do that day is beyond comprehension for most people.

I also think you sort out who your friends are when you deal with a chronic illness. There are people who have disappeared from our lives because they couldn't deal with the challenges that living with MS brings. I know they are the ones that had the problem; not us. I remember a few times Annie would be quite upset at realising how fickle some friendships had become. But on the other hand, we've formed some very close friendships with other people who have been amazingly supportive. They've become our tight support circle and they're invaluable.

The uncertainty is the big thing you struggle with when dealing with MS. It can be anything from uncertainty around disease course through to mundane things like whether there is disabled access or where we can get travel insurance.

I'm a pretty seasoned business person who probably thrives a little bit on crisis management but nothing prepares you for the daily unpredictability of a degenerative disease. And widespread ignorance about MS doesn't help the matter at all.

We get quite good at controlling so many other facets of our life but the changing nature of MS is one of those things that is completely unable to be controlled by the carer, let alone the person living with the disease. I've spent most of my life professionally solving problems and this is one problem I can't solve. And when you attempt to solve it, you're inclined to think that you're doing it entirely alone. I do think that's one thing the various MS societies have done really well; they've created a support network that others can reach out to.

I've never talked publicly about my wife's MS experience or mine as a carer until now because frankly I think it is typical of many people with MS; nothing out of the ordinary. I discussed this interview with Annie. Her comment was MS research probably won't help her but as a mother and grandma, it is vital that our daughters' and grand-kids' generations be helped. MS research offers people with MS, and their carers, the one thing they all cling to – hope for a cure and a better quality of life. I couldn't have put it better myself!

LOUISE MURRAY, HELEN OWENS, KAREN MURPHY AND JAY MCVICKER - FRIENDS

"What I do for her doesn't detract from our friendship. I never wake up and think 'okay, what do I need to do for Jillian today?' But there is an essence of being there to help her with whatever she needs and just generally making sure she knows she's not alone." – Louise Murray.

The following interview was conducted by Channel Nine news reporter Ebony Cavallaro for inclusion in this book. After much consideration, the author felt very strongly that the journey and viewpoint her own friends could share would be important in assisting other people who have friends with MS. At the same time, the author knew she couldn't impartially interview her friends herself and was honoured to have such an accomplished journalist in Ebony Cavallaro assist in the process. The following chapter is a dialogue of their interview.

So how do each of you know Jillian?

Helen: I met Jillian when she became a client of mine at one of the hair salons I own; it feels like I've known Jillian 15 years but it's only actually been six or seven. We really hit it off on a personal level but then Jillian started doing some of my marketing and media work and it got to a point where we were inventing meetings so we could catch up. Needless to say we never got much work done so we stopped pretending to have meetings and just caught up because we wanted to hang out with each other.

Karen: Jillian and I went to high school together. Jillian was a boarder at the school we attended and I was a day girl. The boarders tended to stick together so I wasn't overly close to Jillian at school, but our paths crossed again about four years ago when we were planning a 25 year school reunion. Since then we've gotten to know each other really well, helped each other along the way and simply enjoyed each other's company. We both went through our marriage breakdowns at roughly the same time and I think that has also brought us closer together.

Louise: Karen, Jillian and I all went to school together, but it's only been over the last few years that Jillian and I have become particularly close. I didn't actually make it to our school reunion but a booklet had been produced for the event detailing where everyone was from our year and I realised Jillian only lived a few streets away from me. We caught up for a coffee one day shortly after the reunion and then pretty much every day since! We realised that as adults we had many similar interests so we tend to hang out together and that's a lot of fun. I think we both loved each other's company and it's been such an easy friendship to grow.

Jay: The way that Louise and Jillian connected is very similar to how we connected as well. I think it's part of the typical Teneriffe lifestyle. For an inner city suburb of Brisbane we have built such a tightknit community here and Jillian is a big part of that community. We lived only a few streets from each other and Jillian was a client of our business and our business was also a client of Jillian's. There's not too many degrees of separation between anyone in Teneriffe!

Do you remember how you found out that Jillian had MS?

Jay: It was actually a very confronting situation for me. Jillian was in the throes of a marriage breakdown and I had her property listed for sale. To be honest, her ex-husband had lost the plot a little bit and I was getting regular, abusive phone calls from him about the sale of the property. I know there was a lot of pressure on both of them, and looking back, clearly there was a bit more on Jillian to hold everything together. She called me early one week and casually mentioned that she had lost feeling down the left side of her body and felt like she was getting a bad flu. As each day passed she became a little bit worse until she ended up in hospital on a Friday afternoon. It took a few days before the doctors could work out what was going on; I believe at first they thought she had suffered a stroke.

During this time I had gotten a contract in on her property and I know the terms were what Jillian wanted even though the timing wasn't fabulous. But this is just how Jillian is as a person. No matter what else is going on, if she's got something she wants to achieve she won't let anything stop her. I found myself in a position where I was going back and forth between my office and her hospital bed to negotiate the contract and there came a time where I just wanted Jillian to sit back and focus on her health and nothing else. I couldn't seem to get her to understand that her health needed to be the priority.

She'd be very bossy and declared "No this is what I want Jay. I just want to get this done and finish this chapter of my life."

Despite my suggestions that Jillian should nominate a power of attorney and the protestations that it really wasn't even very appropriate for me to be doing bedside negotiations, she held her ground. In fact it was while she was signing the final contract that she casually told me she'd been definitively diagnosed with MS. She was very casual about the diagnosis from the very beginning but I think she was in a state of extreme shock.

Karen: I think she had so much going on at that time. Just trying to process the marriage breakdown and the ensuing drama that her ex-husband was throwing at her would be enough to break anyone down, but the health issues that unfolded after that were unfathomable. I don't know how she processed any of it. She was battle fatigued, but I could also see a sad resignation within her. When I found out about Jillian's diagnosis I didn't really know how to react and I still don't understand enough about it to comprehend how it must feel. Whereas when she was diagnosed a little later with breast cancer I guess I had more of an understanding of that disease.

But when I found out that Jillian had MS, I didn't really know what to say. In fact I'm sure I had more questions than comforting things to say to her. Jillian is the first person I've known to be diagnosed with MS – at least directly – and so it was all a little bit confronting, especially given that only months before she was running around, living life and getting on with it, albeit going through some pretty tough times.

Louise: My reaction was a little bit different to Karen's in the sense that by the time I had reconnected with Jillian she was already 12 months into the diagnosis. I never went through that stage of shock because I really hadn't known her in her adult years in any other way. Compared to her other friends, I was probably very blasé about everything but I've also had a lot more exposure to various chronic illnesses and disability.

Regardless, it wasn't until I read her first book that I gained a better understanding of MS and how it affected her personally. She actually held off giving me a copy of 'Taking Control' for quite some time. I don't know whether she was deliberately holding off from giving me a copy because she didn't want to open up or whether she was just being slack! But once I had read the book I gained a totally different perspective on the whole situation. For one thing, I hadn't realised how differently MS affects everyone. Literally everyone has a unique story but with a few common symptoms binding them together. But I also felt much more for her after reading it; before that she hadn't really opened up to me and I couldn't get a good understanding of what her life was like.

The funny thing is that upon reconnecting with Jillian a few years back, I sort of forgot that she'd even been diagnosed with MS. Back then she was still running around a fair bit and acting like nothing was going on.

It wasn't until we became very close that she opened up a little bit more about everything. She is very guarded and doesn't divulge much about how she is feeling to anyone. In fact, I rarely hear her talking to anyone about her feelings or emotions or what she is going through.

Helen: I remember finding out that Jillian was in hospital and I telephoned her just to check in. It was then that she told me she had MS and I don't recall being particularly affected by the news. My auntie had MS but I know I didn't compare Jillian's situation with the journey my auntie had gone through. I just remember saying to her 'you'll be right,' because she always is. I wonder if my reaction might have been more emotional if she'd been standing in front of me?

Louise: I can understand your reaction Helen and I think the general lack of awareness around MS leaves us all a little ignorant as to its effects on the people diagnosed and also their families.

Helen: I totally agree with you Louise. But you know what? Jillian has been all right. We know things are getting tougher on her, but she handles it so well and we do forget that she is living with MS most of the time. I know that if I had MS I wouldn't want my friends to be constantly thinking I'm sick.

After I'd had a little more time to process the news myself I still felt confident that Jillian was going to be okay, but I did feel very strongly that Jillian needed to seek out the best setup for herself over the next five to ten years. I wanted to make sure she was in an environment that supported her disability both emotionally and physically. And over the last few years I have seen Jillian strive to create a supportive environment for herself and this greatly comforts me. She'll soon be moving into a lovely new apartment that caters to all her needs and factors in that her mobility is declining slightly. For a while there I was really perplexed about whether she would need to move in with me and I wasn't sure where I would keep her? I just wanted to make sure she was in the best environment.

Jay: I was never scared by the diagnosis because Jillian explained everything to me very succinctly. I think her state of shock forced her to be overly clinical. But I also think she was actually more relieved to know what was going on. She did a lot of research on MS in those early days.

Louise: She is an incredibly pragmatic person isn't she? I think she just went straight into planning mode as a way of coping with the news.

Karen: She always knew she wasn't going to die from MS, so right from the start she set about living life to the fullest and dealing with the situation as best as she could. When Jillian was diagnosed it was right around the time of our school reunion and it was talked about quite a bit. We were all in our early 40s and it made us all a bit reflective of the different dramas we'd weathered in our lives. I'm pretty sure that no one's life turned out the way we thought it would when we left high school. From a selfish point of view I felt my own age a little bit; it made me realise I wasn't bullet-proof. But I do remember feeling angry and also reflecting that Jillian didn't deserve to get MS; there was certainly other people I would have preferred it handed to before her.

Jay: The really confronting part for me was seeing the progression of Jillian's MS over such a short period of time. One month we see Jillian hooning around Teneriffe in her little Porsche, then she's in hospital for an extended period of time and then shortly after that I met with her parents to discuss what sort of apartment she should buy that would cater to her declining mobility.

I could see they were going into damage control and they wanted to organise a more practical apartment for her to settle into. They were talking in terms of accessibility and functionality rather than the things you'd normally talk about in our suburb, such as river or city views and proximity to the restaurants and shopping. They wanted to know if the hallway was wide enough to accommodate a wheelchair and if the tap fixtures were flick mixers so as Jillian could operate them easily.

It was a very confronting conversation to have especially given the Jillian I knew. But when I reflect back, I think all these confronting times we went through made our friendship stronger. Both Jillian and her family opened up a lot to me throughout her diagnosis and it allowed me to be there for her. The support that we give Jillian as her friends is very different to the support that she gets from her family - as it should be. When Jillian and I hang out as friends I simply enjoy her carefree nature and that she wants to enjoy life. She's a pretty easy person to hang out with because she really does value health and life and wants to live her life to the fullest. And her attitude rubs off on all of us.

I didn't know a lot about MS prior to Jillian's diagnosis and it wasn't until I read her first book that I understood a lot more. Reading the stories of how other people were diagnosed and got on with their life was very helpful in shaping my perspective. Like a lot of people, the first thing I thought about with MS was that Jillian would end up in a wheelchair. But I have come to realise that there are a lot of people out there who function very successfully with MS and for extended periods of time, so I wasn't worried about Jillian's immediate future.

Louise: Even though Jillian was a few years into her diagnosis by the time we reconnected, only very recently did it hit me hard how bad the MS might become for her. We had travelled down to Sydney together where Jillian was speaking at an MS Angels function. It was very interesting hearing from some of the scientists about various MS research projects and then Jillian spoke to the group about her own journey with MS and breast cancer combined and how it has shaped her outlook on life.

While I certainly know most of Jillian's story I'd never heard her speak very publicly and honestly about everything she'd gone through. It was a bit eye opening. But even more so the next day when we met a friend of Jillian's who had been living with MS for more than 20 years and was far more progressed in their symptoms. In fact their mobility was greatly affected and this person had to use a rollater to slowly and awkwardly get around. The mother of one of my other friends has had MS for a long time and I'm no stranger to how the disease could take a toll. But seeing one of Jillian's peers so cruelly affected really stunned me. It was my 'holy crap' moment when I reflected how Jillian might also progress with this rotten disease. And similar to Helen, I worry about how we are going to manage Jillian if her mobility declines that badly. And the frustrating thing is that we can't really plan for any of this. Will it happen? How bad will it get? We just don't know... I had a very heavy heart after that Sydney trip. It was from that moment on I had a lot more empathy for her.

Do you ever think about what Jillian's future might hold?

Helen: It's unrealistic not to think about how the disease might progress. She's recently had yet another hospital stint with an MS flare and she doesn't even know what caused the flare or what damage may have been done, so it's difficult for us to know what to do to help her. I find I just take things day-by-day with Jillian, and to be honest we don't know what's going to happen to any of us in life. Really all I can do is be quite mindful of the situation.

Karen: Yes I think when Jillian was in hospital last time I found the whole situation a little bit frightening. It was only once she finally put herself in to hospital that I found out that she'd been alone and very unwell for about 12 hours while the flare built up. Apparently she couldn't even work her phone properly to dial for help. On hearing her story I became quite insistent that she give us a key to her apartment in case anything like that happened again. I think this last flare must have frightened Jillian as well, as she's consented to giving us a key.

But I still can't wrap my mind around how she can go from being reasonably energetic and upbeat one day to being unable to walk, think, or speak properly the next.

Louise: Yes, I've demanded a key as well. I was travelling with Jillian again last week and everything was fine one moment but she was literally smacked down and overcome by a myriad of MS symptoms the next. She'd had a week of being relatively fine and the change in her health within hours was dramatic. Basically she completely deteriorated in front of my eyes. As close as we are I'd never experienced anything like it.

I know she hides away at home on the days that are really bad and shields everyone from what is really going on. I've seen her in hospital after an attack but seeing her decline so rapidly in front of me was very confronting. All I could do was prop her up and support her in getting onto the plane as quickly as possible. She didn't want to make a scene but she was finding it just so difficult to function. It was one painful step at a time and I don't know how she did it but she just kept pushing forward until she was finally on the plane. I guess in her mind there was just no alternative.

Do you consider yourselves carers and what do you think of that term?

Louise: Yes I absolutely consider myself as one of Jillian's major carers. I see her almost daily and make sure she's eating or getting around. Because I live so close I tend to drive her most places she needs to go as she doesn't like to drive very much anymore. But I'm really just doing what any close friend would do and frankly I like that she's letting me help her out a bit more. What I do for her doesn't detract from our friendship. I never wake up and think 'okay, what do I need to do for Jillian today?' But there is an essence of being there to help her with whatever she needs and just generally making sure she knows she's not alone.

About 18 months ago Jillian had a major surgery for her breast cancer and reconstruction and we knew it required a long recovery time. When she was finally released from hospital I asked her to come and stay with me at the beach for a week. As tired as she was I didn't want her lying at home by herself. So she came up to our place and we had a really good time laughing and talking and it was the first time she really opened up about everything that had gone on and how she wanted to get on with her life. I think it was fairly cathartic for both of us. And I feel a lot closer to her because of it. But I don't really bring up much conversation about the MS unless she does.

Jay: In some ways I feel more like a protector than a carer. If we go out together I know she gets really worried about how other people will perceive her when she is using a walking stick. But she doesn't want to become isolated and often pushes herself to go out when she shouldn't. For some reason she feels like she has to apologise to me if she is on a walking stick. Mind you, she still wears ridiculously high heels and teeters along with a walking stick just to show the MS who's the boss!

But I'm her protector in both a physical and metaphoric sense. I feel I'm there to protect her from any negative perceptions of the public and I'm also there to physically support her on her wobbly days.

Louise: I know Jillian gets very frustrated at how invisible MS can be. She finds it hard to explain just how badly and inconsistently she is affected by MS each day. As I mentioned before, one-minute she can look quite normal and the next moment she will go downhill rapidly. I know she should probably use her walking stick more but I think she doesn't want people to think she is any less capable in any way when she is using it. She's an anomaly our Jillian…. she fights so hard for awareness around MS but doesn't want to draw any attention to herself and what she is going through.

Karen: We were both in Hobart a year or so ago and Jillian did use her walking stick quite a bit down there. I think it was because she was in an environment where no one would recognise her. But people would constantly stop her in the street to ask where she got her sticks from. She has quite a collection in different designs and colours. She commented to me how blown away she was that everyone was being lovely about the sticks. I asked her if she expected people to come up and be anything other than nice and she didn't really have an answer to this.

Then there's been a few times I wish to god she had been on her stick, and it all comes back to the invisible nature of MS. A group of us had gone out one evening to a local bar and Jillian was yet again teetering on heels despite suffering vertigo. She really wasn't walking very well but was mortified to think she'd be going to a trendy bar looking like a geriatric (her words, not mine…) on a walking stick, so she refused to use it. She was fairly unsteady and was walking her fingers against a wall to keep her balance. The bar's bouncer saw her looking unsteady and wouldn't let her inside. She explained that she had MS and that she was always off-balance, but the bouncer just looked at Jillian blankly and refused her entry.

I stepped in to explain that she wasn't intoxicated. I'm a qualified lawyer (but don't practice any longer) so my natural tendency is to fight against the injustices. I tried to educate this bouncer and once again he stared at us impassively before finally replying "I just don't give a fuck."

Well, things spiralled a bit out of control after that because it was such a ridiculously ignorant response to a very real situation. I know we all agree that Jillian doesn't like to make a fuss about things but this was one night when we both wanted to stand up for what was right. The bouncer actually asked us for some sort of formal letter or identification that Jillian had multiple sclerosis. I was arguing that they don't really make ID cards stating what sort of disease one has.... He was just being a bit of a smart ass.

This guy threatened to call the police when we persisted in being allowed entry to which I said 'go ahead!' I was so riled up by that point. We weren't doing anything wrong and it was pure discrimination.

So the police arrived and to be honest, they were even worse than the ignorant bouncer. There was a female police officer who immediately took offence to us. By this time, Jillian was actually sitting on a ledge that led into the venue as she had no energy or balance left after arguing. We looked at each other and decided to leave because the police officers were carrying on with more ignorant comments. Anyway, as Jillian got up to leave, she lost her balance and fell backwards and the female copper stepped forward and started reading Jillian her rights!

At that point I was so appalled that I lost it. I went off my nut at the officer. I think the only reason I didn't end up getting arrested myself was because a taxi pulled up in front of us and we had the sense to both jump in and speed away.

It was the first time I'd been confronted with what she must put up with all the time. It was so disgusting and disrespectful. I felt the police were actually being quite abusive in the end. She's damned if she does and damned if she doesn't. She wants to preserve some semblance of her personal style and dignity by not always using a walking stick, but if she doesn't use it, people don't believe she's battling a very serious disease.

Louise: I can certainly understand why Jillian wouldn't want to rely on the stick. I don't care how cool her collection is. I think for her it's maintaining a bit of independence and I'm sure there's certainly some vanity in there as well.

Karen: There's certainly some vanity involved and I get that. She's worked really hard to get to where she is in life and she wants to hold her head high and look good doing it. After her last hospital visit she told me that one of the physio's had started talking to her about perhaps using a wheel chair to get around at crowded events or when her energy is poor. I think Jillian started getting her mind around the notion that needing to use a chair might be a bit closer than she imagined. I pushed a little bit to take her to get fitted for one, even if it meant that the chair sat tucked away in a cupboard until she needed it, but she was still pretty defiant that she wasn't ready.

The day after she was released from hospital for that MS flare she went to a Melbourne Cup lunch. It was that defiance coming out again – she wasn't going to let the MS curb her lifestyle too much! The well-known para-Olympian Karni Liddell was at the same lunch and when she wheeled in, Jillian's eyes lit up. Here was a gorgeous young woman, proud and confident and just happened to be in a wheel chair. I think Jillian got her mind around the concept of a wheelchair from that point.

Helen: My auntie with MS called her support crew her 'Multiple Friends.' It was kind of cool because it was this really supportive posse of friends that all did something different for my auntie; and she made it sound like a fairly exclusive club to get into. They were one tight little group.

**What's your process if you're concerned about Jillian?
What do you do?**

Karen: I've had the others text me if they can't get a hold of Jillian. Sometimes she just goes a bit dark; she maintains radio silence as a way of shutting out the world on the bad days.

Louise: I think most people know how regularly I see Jillian and will call me if they haven't seen her for a few days, just to check that everything is okay.

Helen: I figure that no matter what she's going through she's going to be okay, and if she's not, she'll tell us. She's often more concerned about other people and I think placing her empathy towards others is her way of deflecting what's going on in her own life. But I know she's also getting better at reaching out or giving us a bit of a head's up on how she's feeling. She'll never make a production out of it but she'll tell me when she's ready. Another friend of ours, Antonella, will check on her via text quite regularly and I think Jillian has been able to open up to her a bit and provide a quick yay or nay as to whether she's feeling okay. They've got a good banter going on.

**Have any of you done any specific research on how to support
someone with MS?**

Karen: I Googled it but despite there being so much information from around the world it's all pretty vague. I've found that it depends on the individual and the impact that the MS has on that person. I've never really found any good information and I think we are doing everything that we can do at the moment.

Louise: There is no checklist and even to this day I still forget that Jillian has MS, until something happens. And that's when it really hits you. That episode she had at the airport recently hit me with a big stick. And that's when I realised her attacks were happening far more regularly. I think the MS is really settling in for Jillian.

Karen: I don't think I could even write a checklist of advice for people supporting friends with MS. It's a fairly moveable feast and it's entirely dependent on how MS affects the person and also the type of relationship you have with the person with MS. And I also think that the things I could have supported Jillian with right after her diagnosis are very different to how I can support her now that the disease is progressing a bit more in her. What she was capable of doing then and what she's actually able to do now are two different things. The MS has really made Jillian change her life fairly rapidly, particularly over the last 12 months.

Louise: And she is actually snappier with people.... But I think she's at the stage where she just thinks "Stuff it. If you're pissing me off, I'm going to tell you." She'll often say to me that she just doesn't have time to beat around the bush any more. And I see it coming out more and more. She's become very pissed off that she has MS. Her mindset has really changed on this lately; if she's annoyed with someone or something she'll certainly let them know and I figure it's because the MS lets her know when it doesn't want to play.

Helen: I have no doubt that her tolerance in many areas would have altered quite a bit.

Jay: I don't know that I really know what Jillian needs. Our relationship is a bit like that of a big sister and little brother. I think sometimes it's just being there to provide Jillian with light relief; we have the silliest conversations about ninety per cent of the time. I mean you should hear some of the garbage that comes out of our mouths! She's gotten a lot better at reaching out when she just needs a bit of companionship.

Helen: Yes, she is getting better at reaching out, but I still think it takes her longer than she should to actually reach out. She'll always hear your story first though; I've never known her not to ask what is going on in your life first before she lets you know what's going on in hers.

Jay: Always.

Karen: Yes, she always makes an effort to talk about what's going on in our life rather than talk about her own.

Helen: And then she drops a bombshell about some diabolical thing that's going on with her own health…. I wish she'd stop doing that. I always feel stupid!

Karen: Oh god yes! She always does that. She'll drive 20 min out of her way to have a coffee with you and then after chatting for an hour she'll finally reveal how awful she's feeling that day and it always makes me so cranky that she hasn't let me drive over to see her instead. But I think that Jillian making other people's life a priority and making the effort to get out and about – even on those bad days – is just her way of maintaining some sort of independence and making sure she doesn't get too wrapped up in the drudgery of MS. She just doesn't want to be a burden to her friends or family.

Helen: She definitely wants to be there for everyone else and reminds me of that all the time.

How do you think that the support you give Jillian as friends is different from that support she receives from her family?

Louise: I imagine her parents are more panicked about Jillian than we are. I know even in my own role as a mum I'm constantly concerned about my kids and their well-being. I always think I'd prefer to have something bad happened to me than my kids. Obviously as friends we have a very different relationship with Jillian than she does with her family.

Helen: I think we're there more for Jillian's spirit than for attending to the big picture stuff. I know her family make sure she is fully supported holistically, but I think they rely on us to perform a particular role, and that role is to keep her entertained and keep her spirits up.

Louise: Oh god yes! She still wants to have a lot of fun in life.

Helen: You're right Louise and that's one of the biggest differences between family and friends. Her family are not going to think it's as funny as we do when Jillian falls off a barstool.

Jay: Yes….we don't realise how silly we get sometimes until Jillian's mum comments at our hijinks on Facebook. We always feel so busted! I'm actually waiting for a lecturing phone call from Jillian's parents one day!

Karen: I have actually had her parents question me, believe it or not. They just want to make sure she's not isolating herself and that she is being looked after. But I consider our role is equally as important as the one her family plays.

I know her Mum and sister worry about her terribly. Jillian is pretty open on social media about describing her adventures of living with MS. Her mum or sister will always make very heartfelt little comments, but instead we're all there as friends making really inappropriate and smartass comments.

Helen: I actually think Jillian could survive without our support but she definitely couldn't survive without the support of her family. But she'd be absolutely miserable without our support; we are after all, awesome!

Karen: I liken it to the fact that her family is the foundation of the support network. They're the floors and walls of the building so to speak, but we're the sparkly bits of furniture.

Helen: I know her family help her sustain the things that are really important to her, but we're there to support and bolster her attitude and spirit. I'm not saying we don't add substance in her life but our role is very different to that of her family. I think in life you just like to know that your family is there for you. They don't necessarily even need to do a lot; you just like knowing that they're there.

Louise: I think primarily we're there to give Jillian the emotional support that she needs. And each of us has a very unique relationship with her and we each give her something different. To be honest I'd love a little bit more support from Jillian in the sense of her opening up to us so as we're aware of what's going on. She's such a secret squirrel! She never tells you anything until it's actually happened or bordering on it being too late for us to help her better. And I understand why she tries to hold everything in but I think just a bit more transparency as to how the MS is really affecting her on a day-to-day basis would be really helpful.

Helen: I remember a conversation not that long ago when she was disgruntled with a few people. There was a group of other friends whom had always been in her life but she thought they just weren't there as much for her as she needed them to be as the MS progressed. She didn't need them to be doing anything for her but she just wanted a bit more understanding from them as to what living with MS was like.

I actually questioned her as to if she had reached out to them to explain how she felt. She agreed that she hadn't done much in the way of reaching out to them at all. I then counselled her that if I was on the periphery of her life I would probably find it hard to break into it as well, as she plays everything pretty close to her chest. There's a difference between wanting people to come into your life and allowing them to do so. She needs to give permission to more people to be part of her life.

Can you name a few ways that your own lives have changed from having a friend with MS?

Helen: I'm a lot less worried about structure in my life and I'm certainly more carefree about things. One thing that Jillian has taught me is to calm down and prioritise what's really important. I'm the sort of person who is always being a bit hard on themselves about what they need to achieve but after I've seen what Jillian's been through I've realised that my world isn't going to crumble if I don't get one or two things done and that there's probably more important things than constantly working.

Karen: I'd agree with Helen. But one of the main things I've learnt from Jillian is that simple is good. She has really simplified her life since she's been diagnosed – compared to what it was – and she is far better for it. I just know she is so much happier and more content even though she's had a ridiculous array of health issues to deal with.

Helen: She's re-found her passion in writing and she would never have rediscovered that if it weren't for the changes she had to make in life. She'd still be pottering away, sorting out other people's media problems and feeling utterly miserable with it.

Karen: The MS has actually enabled her to do what she loves as opposed to what she had to do to put money in the bank. And let's face it most of us would love to do what we really want to do instead of what we feel we have to do. Jillian, to her credit, has grabbed the opportunity with both hands.

Jay: Jillian was such a wound up individual prior to her diagnosis. She always had too much on her plate and every aspect of her life brought stress. She was constantly working and would never take time out to chill. In reflecting on the changes that Jillian's diagnosis has brought to her life it has made me realise that there really is nothing more important than your health. I get that we have to do what we have to do to make enough to pay the bills, but it's all for nothing if you don't have your health.

Helen: And this isn't rocket science. We know that our health should be important but we rarely do much about it. It's not until you actually witness the impact of a major health crisis on someone else – and someone so close – that you actually comprehend its significant effect.

Louise: Jillian's situation has changed how I think about my health. It's made it easier for me to clarify what I do and don't want. I was never particularly concerned about growing old but I do want to ensure I'm as healthy as possible as I age. And especially when I see Jillian have her flares, it's particularly confronting and I selfishly think that I don't want to be like that. So Jillian's situation drives me to live as healthily as I can every day. I now eat a lot more organic food and am constantly quizzing her as to all the different health tips she talks about. And I guess my change in attitude has had an impact on my family as well. I have a blended family and it's become really important to me to be as healthy as possible so as I can be there for them. I no longer want to just keep plodding along and hoping everything will be okay. I definitely have a greater sense that I have to take control of my own health, well-being and happiness.

What have you struggled the most with in supporting Jillian through this process?

Jay: I very much struggle with the fact that Jillian doesn't reach out when she needs help.

Karen: I'd agree with that Jay, and just hearing about some of the other flares that Jillian's had but hasn't told me about really annoys me. I'm annoyed and worried that she still isn't letting us in enough.

Helen: She says that she doesn't want to bother us, and I get that, but she needs to know that we want to be there to help and I don't think any of us think we're doing enough to support her.

Louise: I struggle with the fact that she thinks she might be burdening us. I know she doesn't necessarily want to rehash everything that's going on with several different people and thus perpetuating how bad she feels at times, but we need to work on finding a balance where she feels she can confide and we feel we can ask what's going on. I would hate to think that Jillian didn't know she's allowed to pick up the phone and download to us about anything at any time.

As Jillian's support network, why did you want to share your story?

Louise: I got a lot out of Jillian's first book and I know she's a huge believer that real life stories have a powerful way of transforming and informing. So if something we've talked about today can help just one other person, then that's amazing. And I don't think you necessarily have to know anyone with MS to get something out of the books. They're stories that can shape your attitude towards life.

It frustrates me greatly how little awareness there is around MS. We at least know what it stands for but most people would have no idea how it affects a person or what having MS means. I would love to see better awareness around the disease.

Karen: I really wanted to highlight how important it is for someone living with MS to maintain a group of friends away from the support that a family may provide. The interaction with friends – just doing fun and normal things in life – is what keeps you sane.

What's the best piece of advice you can give someone else in helping their friend deal with MS?

Helen: Just to be present. And to encourage everyone to be very open as to what's going on and how they're feeling.

Karen: And to just listen and watch. Be aware that MS is really different to everyone living with it and their needs will be individualised.

Louise: And to first and foremost just be there as a friend and all the other support will just come naturally.

Jay: Just to be available.

***

EPILOGUE

Through working with Jillian to get background research and then interviewing this dynamic group of friends, it really hit home to me how important each of them are in Jillian's life. They are her lifeblood. She talks about each and every one of them all the time and is so grateful for the unique ways each of them provides support. I also know how appreciative Jillian's parents are of the support each of these people gives their daughter. They feel reassured of their daughter's safety and wellbeing just knowing they're around. – Ebony Cavallaro, Journalist

Dear Louise, Helen, Jay and Karen,

They say the most memorable people in your life are the ones who loved you even when you weren't very loveable. And thank goodness for you guys. Without you I'd surely be a quivering mess, no doubt sprawled on some dirty lino floor in a flop house in the outer suburbs of Brisbane...... I simply would have given up.

You feed my soul and nurture my spirit. You're helping me create memories that sustain me through the dark nights. You've all become part of this wild adventure with me and I couldn't imagine a better posse to take it with.

I know I'm a bit of a 'secret squirrel' but I really hate the fact that I might be burdening anyone with anything. I can't help it. It's the way I've been raised and asking for help has been a hard lesson to learn. Slowly but surely – and with your encouragement – I'm learning that leaning on you a little doesn't make me weak. In fact, I'm starting to feel more empowered for it. I think we need a theme song in that respect. (I nominate Karen to sift through the music catalogues but can we avoid the likes of Gloria Gaynor, Beyonce and even Katie Perry to find our theme song...)

You guys really are the best. We've all suffered a few casualties in the friendship pool over the last few years but I'm so grateful that it was you four who were left standing. I know where I stand with each of you, I know I can be myself and I know honesty is the glue that holds us together. And champagne coated love. We also have gallons of that.

You guys mean the world to me and I hope you understand that anything going on in my life is never more important than what's going on in your world and I'm always here to listen, defend or fix what I can.

Writing a letter like this is a bit like an Oscar's speech and I'm going to forget someone or something I need to acknowledge. Two other friends I'd like to make special mention of are Antonella and Ruth. Neither of these two gorgeous girls were interviewed for the book, because frankly they know where the bodies are buried and there's some things we need to exercise discretion on. No seriously, their omission from this interview is not an indication that they are any less special to me. They were probably off doing something more fabulous anyway!

Well the writer in me could ramble for another 1000 words or so but best I wrap this up before it becomes too soppy.

James – I love that within seconds of being in each other's company we are laughing and being silly. But for all that silliness you have given me much sage advice over the years and plenty of guidance. Mwah! Love you!

Karen – Without a doubt I know I can depend on you. How lucky am I to have a friend like that. You have stood up and fought for me and you have pulled me into line when I needed it. I look forward to growing old together but I'm still not going to share a pink mobility scooter with you.

Helen – Ohhhh Snoodle. What can I say? I think a sign of true friendship is when you have a pet name for someone. We both know how rare it is to just 'click' with someone in life. You really have been there for me every step of the way. I love that we can just sit down anywhere, anytime and pour our hearts out to each other. And we're getting better at doing that without the influence of wine. (Oh who am I kidding....)

Louise – Mon ami. I can't imagine how terribly drab my life would be without you. We have developed such an easy friendship and it sometimes scares me how much we can read each other's mind. You are the Grace Adler to my Karen Walker. Or the Patsy to my Eddie. I may draw the line at a Thelma and Louise analogy because neither of us really want to drive over a cliff because of a man... But seriously, you go above and beyond and you influence my life every day. You take such good care of me without realising that the small things help such a tremendous amount. I look forward to so many more amazing journeys with you – the world is our oyster.

Big love, my friends....

Jillian xx

RATU LEWIS - HUSBAND

"All I can remember about that moment were quiet tears. I think they were tears of resignation because Loretta had already figured it out."

M eeting Loretta was fate. We were both fairly typical 22 year olds, except I think Loretta probably had a nicer car than I did. It was back in the mid 90s and I'd successfully interviewed for a job with Sunsuper in Brisbane and was eventually transferred into Loretta's team. To be honest, we didn't get along that well when we first met. She was so professional and capable at her job and I was the guy who asked too many questions. More often than not she would be quite abrupt with me and eventually I just gravitated towards other people within our team.

But a few months after we started working together something changed in our dynamic and we ended up becoming really good friends and eventually dating. Initially we tried to hide our romance from everyone at work, but within a week everyone knew anyway; we couldn't disguise our affection for each other! We moved in together only weeks after we started dating and were engaged about six months after that.

We married in 1997 and both progressed with our careers, climbing the corporate ladder and also accepting transfers around Australia. Eventually kids followed but before that we certainly lived life to the fullest.

About two years ago Loretta started feeling some weird stuff going on with her body. In fact she hadn't felt as well as she normally would for a few months. She was experiencing a range of symptoms – which appeared to worsen when she was exercising – so she chalked everything up to a niggling injury. However, after many months of a continuing and severe fatigue and the fact that these 'injuries' still hadn't settled, a GP referred Loretta to a neurologist for an MRI to rule out anything more sinister. Her MS diagnosis unfolded from there.

The whole time I was a bit blasé to the events. Certainly I was concerned for Loretta's general well-being but it never once occurred to me that this wasn't something that would go away. We're both super-busy people anyway; Loretta was working full time in a management position at Q-Super; I run a business and then we have four kids – William aged 12, Elizabeth who is 10 and twin girls Emily and Lucy who are four. My own business necessitates me attending a lot of events, so between work and the kid's school activities we're over-scheduled people and never had time to stop and think.

Loretta went to that first MRI in 2013 alone but she had a funny feeling as to what the diagnosis might be. She'd read a lot of research leading up to seeing the neurologist and had already drawn her own conclusions. I urged her to just wait and let the specialists do their job because I didn't want her panicking. It had already been a long and drawn out process across four months but once our neurologist had seen the MRI she was able to confirm that Loretta had MS.

All I can remember about that moment were quiet tears. I think they were tears of resignation because Loretta had already figured it out. But it's still shattering to hear the words and have it confirmed. Soon after, the tears turned to devastation as we dwelled on the impact it might have on our life. But then for some reason – maybe it was hope, maybe it was naivety – I thought it really wouldn't have any impact on our lives until we were well into our 60s.

When talking to the neurologist for the first time I remember thinking that she might never experience anything more than the milder symptoms she started off with and that any treatment would halt progression. I guess I was hoping for a status quo.

A lot of the reading I'd done on MS cited that the symptoms worsened as people neared their 60s. I thought we had a great deal of time before we had to really worry – especially where her mobility and balance was concerned. In the meantime we could re-arrange things to manage her fatigue and treatments. In a way, I figured that if she was resting at home then she'd be able to manage the kids and that would allow me to be out with my business more!

And in theory that worked for a while. She would drop the kids to school, rest throughout the day then pick the kids up. Our lives actually became simpler during this time. But about twelve months ago Loretta's symptoms deteriorated again and I started worrying about how much time we would have left to do the things we'd planned.

This was to be a short-lived sentiment however. The unending fatigue had already started to dig in for Loretta. MS can be a strange disease. While I understand the ebbs and flows of her lassitude, Loretta always worries that when she's having a good day (or even a good few hours) people will look at her and think 'well, what's wrong with you? Could it really be that bad?'

The other day we were at a shopping centre and she needed to use a wheel chair. I'd never realised how different it can be pushing a wheelchair compared to a pram. It's significantly heavier for starters and people tend to stop and smile at prams but stare at wheel chairs. It can be quite unnerving. I do worry about what other people think. Loretta is capable of getting up and out of the wheel chair and standing for a while but we use the chair in crowded environments so as she can keep her balance and also conserve her energy. People don't understand this and I'm sure they think it's some type of fake illness. Maybe I'll stop worrying about people's attitudes one day, but for now it's an odd experience. I imagine it would be more difficult for Loretta to reconcile herself to it though.

Loretta decided she wanted to remain at work as long as she could. She simply loved her work and she was just so good at it. And it was a very important form of independence for her. I think particularly given that we'd spent a fair proportion of our careers working together before I started my business, her remaining at work as long as possible was her way of having a separate identity. But she still worried a lot whilst at work. She had an excellent rapport with her boss so decided to inform him about the diagnosis more-or-less immediately. I think she was dreadfully worried that her peers would perceive her as being weak. I knew she didn't have anything to worry about and naturally her colleagues were tremendously supportive but I can understand the fear involved with telling people you've got MS or that you have to start giving up things in your life because of it.

We told Loretta's parents and siblings the day we found out and I also told my brother straight away as I work with him in the business. We then started telling our staff informally over the next few weeks. I'm pretty open about everything and I thought it would be easier on everyone if they understood what was going on. Nearly everyone knew someone else with MS but they didn't really know what MS was or the ways it can effect a person. They had a lot of questions about Loretta's symptoms and how she was dealing with it. And surely, whenever there was a television or magazine feature about MS everyone would let me know. And if someone reads about a new cure or treatment they are very good (and forward) about suggesting we should get onto it straight away!

I didn't really have a strategy on who should find out when, but I found myself telling the people I work with before I'd even told my mates. When I look back on it now, I think deep down I knew it was going to be harder to tell those closer to me. At the time I remember feeling as if something was broken in our life and I didn't want my friends to see that in me. I didn't want them to be burdened with what we were facing. We weren't used to asking for help or having anyone put themselves out for us. But that's been something that has changed more recently and we're getting better at accepting help.

When you've constantly got people asking if they can help it can have the opposite affect to what is intended. Sometimes I would irrationally think the offers of assistance were an indication that people didn't think I could cope. But I'm recognising that my attitude towards help is gradually changing, it's just taking time. I think it's always going to be hard to accept help – it's a matter of pride – but as things become more difficult to manage by myself, I understand the value of what's being offered and the sheer necessity in accepting assistance.

The kids' schools have been overwhelmingly supportive. They've just started dropping us a few meals a week as their way of helping. It's just such a lovely and supportive thing for the school community to do.

And then there's the unsolicited advice that we're constantly offered…. generally about revolutionary diets or a certain lifestyle we should be living or retreats we should attend. I do find it frustrating but I realise the advice is coming from a good place. My standard response is to nod and thank the person.

Both before and after her diagnosis, Loretta did a great deal of reading about MS and has subsequently changed to a vegan diet. She's also undertaken a variety of treatments as we try to figure out the one that suits her best, but frustratingly her symptoms are ever-evolving. It's been difficult to pin down any particular treatment that will work for her.

Throughout all this time I was being a typical male and trying to come up with solutions. I just wanted to solve everything. I immediately thought we should move from Brisbane back to Melbourne. The cooler climate would be more comfortable for Loretta and I feel more at home there. I also wanted Loretta to stop work immediately. But really I just wanted to do anything at all to support her. During these early days I never ever lost it in front of her but I would get quite emotional when I was alone.

It was only about six months after her diagnosis that work started taking a huge toll on her. The fatigue was becoming unmanageable and unpleasant and I think the stress of managing the work and fatigue was causing additional fatigue. It was a vicious circle. I could see the price that Loretta was paying but I didn't want to be the one to suggest taking away something that gave her such a sense of worth.

The eventual process of Loretta leaving work made the MS even more real. People started asking a lot more questions but it was also the transition to a new stage of life after nearly 20 years of working that made us both stop and pause.

It's now been two years since the diagnosis and I take everything a day at a time. I don't consider that I have a support network. My friends and family are wonderful but at this stage I don't want to unload on them. There's more value in me just getting out with my friends and relaxing, but I don't necessarily want to talk to them about MS or the challenges we're facing. I find it incredibly difficult to talk about the worry I'm feeling. It's something I hold in. I'm probably a fairly typical male in that regard. I have a few female friends that I find I can talk to about this stuff more easily, as women tend to ask more questions conversationally, but male conversations don't really work to that dynamic, so as a general rule I don't unload to anyone at all.

Maybe it's also because I get a lot of energy from the people around me and I don't want that to change. I publish a magazine so I can often be speaking with people late into the night. I don't see myself using it as a distraction but rather as remaining connected to the real world.

We had always wanted to travel extensively. Now we've just moved everything up a bit. We took off to New York for a week on the spur of the moment and we do have a different concept of time to what we previously did. MS definitely makes you contemplate how you spend your time – not just with your partner but also with family and friends. Now it's about making sure I enjoy my life and cherish time with my kids and wife.

Living with MS in the family has certainly had an impact on my working life as well. I've been making some choices with regards to my business so that I can prioritise my family. I used to always think 'there'll be time for that later' but now I know there may not be. And when everything is cruising along in life nicely, we forget that a full life is actually not a long time. We're both in our 40s now, but that's about half way through a lifespan!

Two years ago I wouldn't have even dreamed I'd be making the decisions that I'm making now. Back then my primary focus was turning the business into something massive. My only family focus was to get the kids through school. Our financial dynamic was also different prior to Loretta's diagnosis. She made a strong income in her role and this allowed me to build my publishing company and put all the profits back into the business. I've always wanted a hands on role in my kids' lives, which was one of the driving reasons for starting the business, so as I could have that flexibility.

Loretta was an incredibly fit and active person – and particularly with four kids she handles a lot. But now to see her needing to rest after a mere 10 minutes of walking, it's upsetting. I try not to reflect on it too much. I simply go into carer mode. I've only gotten frustrated that she needs such frequent rests a few times and it's mainly around situations that involve the kids. One of my biggest concerns is making sure the kids still feel like they're getting everything out of life and spending quality time with their mother.

And to be honest, helping the kids deal with the MS is a bit of a struggle. It pulls at both our heartstrings when the twins tell someone that 'mummy's sick.' Our 12 year old son shows such tenacity and has already decided he wants to become a doctor so as he can research MS; he's even come up with some ways he can cure it and I encourage him to keep thinking outside the square – you never know where the cure might come from! And perhaps his desire to create a cure is his own way of taking control of this situation. It's his way of contributing. He might only be 12 but he's already got the male psyche of wanting to 'fix' things. We're keeping an eye on all of the kids. I know our son discusses it with his mates and I'm glad he's got an outlet. We've also made sure his teachers know the situation so they can be aware of any support he may need. I'm hoping that by having everyone involved we're creating a great safety net from the start.

William actually does an awful lot to help out around the house, from helping out with chores through to looking after the two smallest girls, he's really stepped up. And while it's fabulous to have this help I am concerned that he's missing out on the necessary parts of growing up. I want him to feel like a kid too.

Even though William outwardly appears to be the strongest, I think the lifestyle adjustments have been the hardest on him because he's witnessed his Mum go from being a strong career-woman to a vulnerable figure, constantly battling fatigue. He's very aware that stress can affect her badly, possibly even setting off a round of spasms in her. The Catch 22 is that William is a teenager and as teenagers are prone to do, he has his fair share of arguments with us. But more often than not he'll now just give up and walk off mid-argument, so as not to cause Loretta any stress. I don't want anyone arguing but I also don't want him to lose his character or voice.

But then Elizabeth, our second eldest daughter – she doesn't tell anyone that her mum has MS. She's very quiet about it and has a tendency to shut herself away.

Observing how Elizabeth deals with all this can be tough at times. I personally feel that all I can do is stand back and watch how she reacts to things. I guess I'm monitoring the situation without imposing my beliefs onto her. She's at that age where she does need a lot of attention and re-assuring and perhaps even if Loretta didn't have MS she'd still be quiet and introspective. But I get a sense she's holding a lot in because when she does finally ask us a question, it will be about something that happened weeks ago. I can tell she's thinking deeply about everything that's going on. I'm pretty careful to casually check in on her every day; just allowing her to know that we're there for her and ready to talk when she wants. I guess I want her to feel safe discussing anything when she needs to.

But it's quite interesting to see how the younger girls react to the situation. They were both 3 years old when Loretta was diagnosed, so they really don't know their mum to be any other way. There's been times when Loretta was in the kitchen – say preparing our evening meal – and her spasms might overwhelm her and she'll end up on the floor. The girls would simply walk into my office and nonchalantly let me know that 'mummy is on the floor,' before going back to watching TV. Or if she passes out from fatigue while reading them a bedtime story, one of them will always come and find me and let me know to put mummy to bed. I'm glad that Loretta's symptoms aren't alarming to them; I guess it's that ebb and flow of finding our new wave of 'normal.'

Loretta and I have worried that our children might get MS. We're not consumed by the thought but it's a little niggle in the back of our collective mind that's hard to ignore. There's no logical way to deal with these thoughts other than to try to put them out of our mind. Having said that, I still remain a little sensitive to any abnormalities my kids are experiencing. Are they getting clumsier? Can they see properly? I particularly monitor William because out of all our children he reminds me of Loretta the most. Anyone who's been diagnosed with MS knows that it's rarely something you can see coming and that's a really scary thought. I don't want any of my kids to have it, but on the flip side, how could I even stop it if they were susceptible?

Life at home can be quite lonely at times. Even though Loretta is there physically, she's not always mentally present. The exhaustion she experiences is just so gutting. I want her to rest and conserve energy, but it's very isolating and something I've found hard to cope with. I don't want to talk to anyone about it, because that would just appear selfish, but whenever I do speak to others, they are always primarily concerned with Loretta. And I understand she is the focus, but you can also experience a little bit of loss of self in this whole process. When I'm lonely I'll just keep busy with chores or talk to my writers and keep them on track with their work. I guess I find it easier to busy myself with mundane tasks.

One of the things we loved doing was watching the TV together at night. Our ritual was to get the kids to bed then turn the TV on at about 9.30pm and watch programs together. It was our time. But I found that when Loretta was in hospital or unwell at home, I'd very rarely turn the TV on. It just didn't appeal to me if I couldn't do it with her.

Also when the kids were asleep I would feel terribly alone and I didn't like it; I didn't like it at all. In the silence of those nights my mind couldn't help but drift to darker places. 'How long does Loretta actually have left?' I'd wonder..... When we'd had conversations about death in the past – prior to her diagnosis – we had both agreed that I was the one who was meant to go first. Sometimes I feel like we've been forced to rewrite our operating manual. And I guess that's not so bad, especially if we're rewriting it with clearer focus on what's really important. She's my best friend so I want to do anything possible to help her.

***

I've found the treatment regime very frustrating – especially when our neurologist is telling us things like 'I haven't ever encountered this situation before.' I feel like everything is just trial and error at the moment; that we're holding out for some treatment to work. I feel like they're using my wife as a guinea pig and that makes me very mad. I do worry that some of the medication she's on is making her feel worse than the disease it's meant to be treating.

We've had instances (particularly when Loretta has been visiting the specialists alone) that certain specialists made her feel like all the pain she's experiencing is in her head. It was even suggested at one point that a psychologist might be the more suitable specialist than a neurologist. Luckily we have an excellent neurologist who definitely confirmed that my wife's symptoms were quite real and frightening and certainly physical, not psychological.

My faith sits firmly with traditional Western medicine, but it can still be frustrating. When I read about how people have healed themselves through things like diet and meditation I think that's great but I keep it in perspective because it's still such a small amount of successful cases compared to how Western medicine is faring.

One of the biggest frustrations I experience is how disparate the information is surrounding MS. You really have to manage the information flow and sources yourself. And there's a lot to manage. It's not a case of lack of information, its more finding the time to manage the sheer amount of it. It's like having another job. And a great deal of the information we find is purely coincidental too. I remember perusing one of the MS society websites and casually coming across a statistic that explained how x amount of dollars fundraised would pay for handrails to be fitted at x amount of houses. It never dawned on me that there might be people or organisations that could help with simple things like that. I thought it was purely our responsibility to take care of it.

I guess one of the biggest concerns is that I just don't know what to ask. I'm sure if I knew what questions I wanted to ask I'd be able to find the appropriate person or organisation to assist me, but there's no guidebook for MS and it's extremely difficult to understand what you're meant to know.

So we find ourselves relying tremendously of the information our neurologist gives us. You have to feel comfortable with that person's ability and also the way that they deliver the information and options.

Loretta has asked me before whether I thought she'd brought the MS onto herself. She was considering whether our lifestyle and the way we lived might have contributed to her diagnosis. Firstly, I vehemently disagree that the way Loretta has lived her life has contributed to her getting MS but I also don't believe you can go through life wondering if you'd done something to cause a disease like MS.

We did have quite an active and social lifestyle. We've certainly been to our fair share of events and parties but I'm now exceptionally glad we did this. Life at the moment is not a party, so I'm glad we lived it up while we had the opportunity. I know Loretta will have more good times and if there's one thing living with MS has taught us, it's to grab those opportunities when you're able to.

When you're caring for someone else with MS it's really important to try and take some time for yourself. Our support role bears a different dynamic to that of the person living with the disease and there's a lot to manage and process. Taking time for yourself needs to be an ongoing process. Ensure you maintain your own sense of identity – your own thoughts – away from the life with MS.

I can't lie to you, but there's times when I get thoroughly over the fact that our life has become all about MS. We're so early into the diagnosis and working out the answers, so I know we won't always be so consumed by it, but for now I find myself becoming quite sick of talking about it.

My form of escapism is attending business functions. I'm invited to a lot of events via my publishing company and I might not spend a lot of time at each event, but I really love the outlet they provide. And Loretta has indicated she likes having some time to herself when I go out. I think it's important for everyone to maintain a sense of individuality and independence and remove yourself from the MS bubble regularly.

I can see how it would be easy for people to let the pressure of living with a chronic illness get to them. Without some avenue to let off steam it would be so damaging to the relationship but also your personal health. This rings true whether it be the person diagnosed or their significant other.

Maintaining your own health is also terribly important. In the times when Loretta has been unwell and I've stopped looking after myself to give her my full attention, I've noticed how quickly I've worn myself out. I had stopped exercising, stopped eating healthily, not gotten adequate rest and let stress get to me. All this took its toll quite quickly and I wasn't much use to anyone. Simply put, we can't afford for both of us – particularly as parents – to be unwell.

And as hard as it might be, it's a much more fulfilling journey to always be supportive of your loved one living with MS.

Know what you're dealing with so as you can be comfortable with the decisions you need to make. I have learned to trust my gut feelings more and more. Loretta is switched on and we tend to agree on just about everything anyway, so I'm lucky. I guess we both agree on the greater strategy of dealing with MS at this stage. The only thing we've ever really butted heads over is the mobility issue. Recently, she expressed very strong feelings about purchasing a wheelchair.

In fact, Loretta's mum went out and bought a wheel chair when she was first diagnosed. I thought it would be something that Loretta and I would do together though, which I guess is another example of me not wanting to relinquish control.

It's really hard to picture your wife in a wheel chair, but Loretta has a way with words and the conversation became more about safety than an admission of loss of mobility. I'm certainly not embarrassed pushing her in a wheelchair but I just don't like seeing her like that. I still struggle with the way that other people react when they see my wife in a wheelchair. I've put the wheelchair in the garage because I don't want to look at it. To be honest, I even put her walking stick away when she doesn't need it, because I just don't want to see it.

I guess a small part of me has been in denial since the moment I found out Loretta had MS. I didn't want to give up hope that everything was going to be alright and I certainly didn't want to give in to the devastation. I just couldn't imagine that her mobility would decline as quickly as it has.

And then the denial was replaced by anger. I didn't like seeing what the MS was doing to my wife one bit. I don't think I ever confided in Loretta but for a while there I found myself being very angry at anything to do with changing our lives. We had to move and look for a new house and I simply didn't want to. I just wasn't ready.

And when there wasn't the anger, there was deep sadness. Over the last two years I have found myself letting the tears flow while I'm driving. It must just be my way of emotional release. I remember arriving to pick the girls up from kindy one afternoon and their teacher grabbed me as I was leaving and said their board had voted to waive the fees that semester so we could take a holiday. It was such a kind thing to do and I kept my tears in check until I got back into the car, then let loose! And other times the tears would just be upon me before I realised what was happening. I found it really hard to let the emotion out. It wasn't a comfortable thing for me to do at all. There were times when I thought my head was going to explode. There's so much information to take on board, so many things in life to consider and then on top of that, dealing with the emotional adjustments.

The other thing that most people wouldn't realise about MS is that you can kiss your time management and organisational skills goodbye. A chronic illness such as MS doesn't care how organised you are or what you have planned.

There were times I could barely think straight with everything I had to process but I knew I just had to take care of the essential things each day. Get the kids ready and off to school, make sure they were fed and looked after and making sure Loretta was okay. But everything else was a jumbled mess.

It's taken me over two years to get back on top of things and feel mildly organised again. I'm a self-confessed control freak but I now realise that you just have to remain flexible and open to anything happening....or not happening.... I've certainly become more laid back and capable of letting go of things.

The fatigue may be the more sinister symptom that Loretta experiences, but when my wife lies down to rest she looks beautiful. However the rollaters, the walking stick or the wheelchair are all visual reminders of what's happened. This is not how we saw our life unfolding.

I go through stages where I'd dearly like to run away from all of this. I want to bundle Loretta up and hide from everything for a month or two. We both get so tired of the stress of MS; there's no respite from the thoughts it brings. I can't help but wish that everything would go back to being normal again.

My darling Ratu,

I am so fortunate to have you, you have been by my side for nearly 20 years. We have been through some pretty rough times over the years. Mental escape artist pets, having our first home broken into, losing our first baby to a late miscarriage, extended house guests, horrible landlords, dodgy builders, dodgy investments, double mortgages and at times worrying how bills were going to get paid. We have gotten through all of life's challenges together and have been the stronger for it. MS is just the latest messed-up hurdle in our life. I am so sorry that it is here to stay.

I know that you keep your emotions in – you always have. And that was difficult to deal with after my diagnosis when we really needed to talk. I was very self-involved while I trying to come to terms with things, strongly using it as my own version of denial; it was hard to see how much you were hurting too. I am so sorry I wasn't there for you. We are always a team but we had to grieve differently, I guess.

I am so grateful for the life we had prior to MS. Our friendship, careers, friends, the things we have done and of course our beautiful children. I can't put into words how much it meant going to New York just after my diagnosis. I literally felt on top of the world! At that point I was still very fit, felt great about myself and had just been rewarded for one of the biggest achievements in my career. It is a memory I will cherish forever.

I know my health has gone pear-shaped since then. You were very understanding and supportive when it got to the point where I couldn't function at work and I started struggling at the gym. It was a very stressful and frustrating time and you put up with a lot of tears and emotion while I went through the process of losing my career and my fitness. Then the spasms started. I honestly don't know how you managed the kids, the business and me in hospital for weeks while the doctors were trying to sort that out.

I appreciate all the things you do for our family. I know that *getting the kids off to school in the morning is a huge effort and you do most of that while I'm only semi-conscience and not much help. Dinner time is even worse. I feel so useless.*

The impact MS has had on all of us has been life altering. While I struggle with fatigue and almost daily spasm attacks, MS has brought us closer together as a family and I am so grateful that it means we spend more time together. You have always been my best friend and I love hanging out with you. Our priorities have completely changed for the better - focussing on each other, creating fun memories with the kids and planning cool holidays. I think we are more appreciative of the things we do have and the amazing people around us.

We have always had a saying that when things are tough, we don't forget what's important. Remember baby, it is still "you, me and us." Not you, me and MS.

I Love you.

Loretta

ADAM MATTINGLY - BROTHER

"Before Katie's diagnosis I would often feel like anything I started in my life wasn't really that important. But suddenly I had a new sense of purpose."

Adam Mattingly is nothing if not a passionate advocate for raising awareness around the need for greater MS research. By day Adam is a keen negotiator for his family's Teflon recycling business, where he sits as vice president. But off the clock, his fashion label Atom Willis claims all his attention in Adam's non-negotiable bid to find a cure for MS.

***

My big sister Katie was diagnosed with MS about nine years ago. I see that Katie's coping technique is to live this super-human life. That's how she appears in my eyes – completely super human. But I know she takes this approach because she feels she doesn't have time to waste or dwell on the bad stuff. And when I get sad, I always bring myself back to the thought of the amazing work that she's doing. She's getting out there and shaking things up when it would have been completely understandable for someone to crumble.

I'm part of a close-knit family. My mother and father live in Houston, Texas, not far from my sister Katie, her husband and two kids. My older brother also lives close by and he has four kids. There's never a shortage of 'uncle duties' for me to undertake!

I grew up in the family business. My grandfather started a gasket company in Houston, which my dad eventually took over. A little over 20 years ago he received an enormous order for parts to be manufactured in polytetrafluoroethylene, better known as Teflon. He had never really worked with Teflon up to that point – back then, it was predominantly used in cookware. After the job was finished he found himself with a lot of Teflon material left over; he didn't want to waste it so he found a way to recycle it. It wasn't until the 1990's that the recycling technique for the material was refined, so it was definitely a niche market.

Eventually recycling ended up becoming our primary function. In a modern-day application, Teflon parts are far superior; they're studier and more durable. In fact, if it were to rain acid, the Teflon parts would survive. When I was younger I really didn't want to go and work for my dad but as soon as I started in the family business I found I really enjoyed it. I'm now the vice president of the company and it's actually a pretty interesting industry.

Business saw me travelling to Korea frequently and I was on a trip in 2010, not long after my sister Katie had been diagnosed with MS. This trip was to be the serendipitous occasion that led me to creating the Atom Willis brand. I had been looking for a lambskin jacket for some time; a friend of mine had found the perfect jacket but paid about $1200 for it, and that was on sale! His jacket set the bar so high and I could never find a match for it. But then on this particular trip to Korea I stumbled upon a guy who owned a clothing factory and produced private label collections for people. Within his showroom I found several jackets within five minutes that I would want to buy and wear.

My brain went into overdrive and next thing I'm asking about customising the design slightly and how to order one hundred of the jackets. By the time I left the store, I knew I was on the path to creating a line that would ultimately contribute to finding a cure for my sister's disease.

Atom Willis is a lambskin leather jacket collection for men. Artisan leather workers create each style with a button-in or out hoodie and a removable, pinstripe and rabbit fur vest. In addition, every jacket has an embossed Atom Willis nickel plate inside the jacket with a serial number that the buyer can register with us. If the jacket is lost it can be returned via Atom Willis to the owner and a portion of every jacket sale goes into the Brass Family Foundation, an organisation started by my sister and her husband.

Over the past four years I've been slowly creating brand awareness and building the business. I'm essentially juggling two jobs but it's still enormously fun. Maybe it's because I know that the success of Atom Willis will directly and positively impact Katie's life.

I worked away on creating Atom Willis for over a year before I finally told Katie and the rest of my family what I was doing and why. I didn't want to tell Katie until I actually had one of my jackets that I could give to her. I'll never forget how big my head was after the first samples arrived. Up until that point I could only dream that they would come back as I had pictured them. The factory making the jackets had initially looked at me like I was insane when I asked for purple stitching as a feature, so I was a little nervous about how they would look.

The day the samples arrived at my office I snuck into the bathroom to check them out; still no one at work or home knew what I had been doing outside my 'day job.' The jackets were beyond amazing and at that point I phoned my parents and I told them about Atom Willis.

In the meantime I had hired a camera crew to come and produce a small movie for the Atom Willis website. I had no idea how to launch a brand or a website so making a short film seemed like an idea with impact. I wasn't completely sure I wanted to reveal in the film that the proceeds from jacket sales would benefit MS research. I think I may have still been a bit uncomfortable with what I was doing. Not because of any stigma surrounding MS but because I hadn't yet talked to Katie about my project.

The film producers urged me to include the purpose of Atom

Willis, knowing that a call to the greater good would provide the edge we needed to stand apart from other designers. Finally I had to come clean with Katie. I went to see her one afternoon and explained what I'd been up to. Coincidently that day she'd received the results of a MRI scan. Up until that point she was convinced that her MS hadn't progressed at all, but with tears she told me the neurologist had confirmed that she had more lesions forming on her brain.

"Do it Adam! We need all the money we can get to find a way to cure this disease," she exclaimed after I told her all about Atom Willis. And from that moment on she's been one of my greatest supporters.

My brand stands for something I believe strongly in and while it may not appeal to everyone, the brand's direction and image is something I'm passionate about preserving. I hate MS. This is the root of our campaign. There is no way we are ever going to cure disease if we are cutting budgets for disease research. In my opinion, researchers should never even have heard of the word 'budget.'

***

Katie's diagnosis was a slow process. She was about 33 when she started experiencing issues with vision and dizziness. At the time she was carrying her first child so thought the issues were simply part of the pregnancy. When the symptoms persisted she consulted two different doctors and both speculated she had MS.

She found it difficult to describe what she was feeling but she knew enough to know it wasn't normal. To be honest, I think our family was initially in denial at the thought it might be something as life-changing as MS and it wasn't until Katie consulted a third specialist in New York City that we finally started grasping what was going on. It was this specialist who explained that the disease is not so clear cut and that it presents differently in everyone and certainly has a different disease course across individuals.

There was a lot of waiting and confusion during this time. Katie told me it was all pretty scary, a bit like anything in life that you're not expecting. Ultimately she knew it would be something that would change her family's life forever.

When I first found out that Katie had MS I was overwhelmed with fear. She's my only sister. At the time I knew very little about the disease but set my mind to finding out as much as possible so I could understand the symptoms and help her.

Katie and her husband AJ started the Brass Family Foundation, which was formed to develop a number of philanthropic activities. One night they were having dinner with their neighbour Bill Perkins. Conversation swung around to the research work of Dr Stephen Hauser, Chairman of UCSF Neurology Department. He had speculated that MS is not genetically passed on but environmental.

Coincidentally, my uncle had seen Dr Hauser speak at a recent event and queried the doctor about his research.

"Doctor, would the world have ever have known this ground-breaking fact if it were not for private funds?"

"Never," replied Dr. Hauser.

Katie, AJ and Bill Perkins were appalled by the fact that MS research simply wasn't finding the cure for MS. They were convinced that with the strong funding and collaborations, something could be done.

And from that conversation the Brass Family Foundation, together with Bill Perkins and Small Ventures USA, raised $1.2 million over 12 months and eventually underwrote a genetic research study in conjunction with Dr. Hauser.

The study, led by Dr Hauser in 2009/10, cited compelling evidence that some powerful non-heritable, environmental factor likely plays a key role in the development of multiple sclerosis. The findings result from the most advanced genomic analysis ever conducted on identical, or "monozygote," twins where one sibling has multiple sclerosis and the other does not. It received worldwide attention from the science and medical fields and was featured on the cover of Nature Magazine, the world's most highly cited interdisciplinary science journal.

The finding does not mean that genes do not play a role in the disease. In cases where one identical twin has MS, there is a 30-percent increased risk that the identical sibling also will develop the disease. In cases where a non-identical twin or other sibling has the disease, there is an increased risk of nearly 5 percent.

The study was the first to examine all three levels of a human genome at the same time, giving the first full picture of a living genome. As far as what environmental factor(s) could be playing a role in multiple sclerosis, the scientists did not speculate in their paper. The most prominent theory in the field is that a viral infection triggers the immune reactions that initiate the disease; Epstein-Barr virus is considered the most likely culprit.

If this were the case, each person's unique genetic make-up would influence the body's immune reactions and determine whether they would lead to the disease. While no viral trigger for MS has been confirmed, several genetic risk factors have been identified. Other current hypotheses include vitamin D deficiency brought on by a lack of exposure to sunlight and smoking. [1]

Dr Hauser went on to receive the prestigious Charcot Award in 2013. The Charcot Award recognises lifetime achievement in MS research and it is given once every two years by the MS International Federation.

***

I was living in Los Angeles when Katie was diagnosed. She was settled in Houston, where my parent's also live, but they still decided to move a bit closer again to Katie. I guess in those early days no one knew what to expect with how the MS might progress. But thankfully the MS has remained reasonably stable and she hasn't needed much assistance from any of us. I guess I see my role in Katie's life as that of any regular brother; I'm there simply to love her, support her and cheer her on and ensure that her life remains great.

The strange thing about starting Atom Willis is that I've found something I'm so passionate about creating, which wouldn't have eventuated if Katie hadn't been diagnosed with MS. But I can't help but think my passion comes as a weird cost.

Before Katie's diagnosis I often felt anything I started in my life wasn't really that important. But suddenly I had a new sense of purpose. I know my parents don't like me getting too distracted from the family business, but as far as the fashion label, they haven't actually told me to stop doing it in the four years I've been developing it. And my sister has never asked me to remove her name from my website; in fact she always tells me how proud she is of what I'm doing. And that really is the best feeling ever.

However, I feel very frustrated at times that I can't do more. I see lots of smaller fundraising efforts happening everywhere and while I know it all adds up, I can't help but think we need some massive donations and a tremendous groundswell to really make great strides with MS research. It drives me crazy and I just don't know what to do.

Katie is amazing. She's incredibly active, both with her kids and philanthropically. She always has something on the go and truly lives life to the fullest. Katie's foundation has raised a substantial amount of money over the years but she's a lot like me. She doesn't necessarily want the attention and accolades. She just wants to get on with it.

And while we're very close, I'm not her girlfriend. We don't have that sort of rapport where we talk all the time about everything that is going on in life. And I get the sense that she doesn't tell me things about the MS because she doesn't want me to worry. But then I'll see her being strong and coping with all her symptoms without any apparent difficulty – and I've seen her go from a really bad MRI to a good MRI – so I can only believe that she's hanging in there strongly. And if she wasn't, I don't think she'd tell anyone in the family anyway.

Sometimes I don't feel like I really know what's going on with Katie's health and that's very frustrating. But I know she's living her life in a really big way. She's such a crusader and so committed to raising MS awareness and I don't think that leaves a lot of room for vulnerability.

So I guess my role in Katie's life is make sure she knows I'm there. We text constantly but it's lots of short little texts showing a lot of love. Maybe that's enough – for her to know that she's loved and supported unconditionally.

But I really feel for Katie. I know she's being strong for her two kids and it's hard on our entire family just not knowing what the future will bring. She can be as strong as she wants but that won't necessarily stop the MS from attacking her.

I feel hope for Katie but I also feel helpless. And I think those duelling emotions have made me a better person. I can now see that most people go about their day as if they have all the time in the world but Katie has made me realise that life holds far greater priorities.

I can't even imagine what Katie goes through and because of that I could never complain about anything. I'd certainly never complain in front of her. And it comes back to recognising your priorities in life. The things I might have been upset about years ago when I was younger are just so insignificant now compared to what she's going through. When I think of my sister I think of someone who's just so special to me and this is one small way I can honour that.

And that's another way my sister's diagnosis has changed my life. I've learned to love a lot more. That fact I know without even having to think too hard about it. When I think of my brother, I think 'Oh yeah, he's cool,' but when I think about Katie this huge wave of emotion sweeps over me. She holds a very special place in my heart. And that familial love then just makes me love my brother more anyway. My mum is really strong too but I can tell she's wanting to die inside because of what Katie is going through. At the end of the day I guess we all just lean on each other for support without making a big fuss about it.

It's really hard to know tangibly how living with someone with MS has changed my life but I just know that everything has done a 180. Everything in my life is different now. I'm driven by my need to find a truth in MS research. As I say in the film I made for Atom Willis,

"Today there's endless truth available. Don't listen to CNN, don't listen to NBC, listen to yourself; occupy your head."

References:

1.   Excerpt from Nature journal: http://tinyurl.com/kt7o4ag

IAN BROOK - HUSBAND

"Our guiding principle is to enjoy life and not sweat the small stuff.
We now firmly understand that life is not a dress rehearsal.
We're not sitting around practicing life....this is the only shot you get."

My wife Regina had been having horrendous headaches for many weeks. In fact, she'd probably been having them a lot longer but didn't tell me because she tends to keep that sort of stuff to herself. Looking back and knowing what I know now, I reckon Regina had lived with MS for at least a few years.

She was also experiencing some tremors and ticks at night but it was those headaches that finally drove her to the doctor. It was hardly shocking that he put them down to work stress. At the time – about 4 years ago – Regina was the administration assistant to the deputy principal at a major school in Brisbane. I was imploring Regina to give up her job if it was that stressful but she would always moan that she had to keep working; deep down I knew she gained a tremendous amount of satisfaction from her role, so I didn't push it too much. The crisis point came though when Regina started visiting a doctor twice a day because of the pain the headaches were causing. The doctors just kept telling her to try different things and take different medications but nothing eliminated the headaches.

Then one night she had a bit of palsy in her face. I wanted to take her to the hospital immediately but she refused and by the next morning it had gone away anyway.

There was all these little symptoms happening all over the place and while they were a minor concern to me, it was when she started losing control of her legs that I became very worried. The first time it happened she'd taken the car out but had to pull over because she couldn't control her legs enough to drive home. She telephoned me distraught and in tears because she didn't know what was going on and if she'd ever be able to drive again.

Not long after, she was explaining her frustrations to colleagues at work when one of them took her aside and said what she was describing sounded similar to a neighbour of hers that had been diagnosed with MS.

That night Regina and I were discussing the comment and she jumped on Dr Google and immediately found a checklist of symptoms. As we went down the list we realised she was ticking an awful lot of boxes. The next day we went back to the doctor again – newly armed with this theory – and demanded that Regina be checked out for MS. He initially started to reject the theory but then something weird happened. He started looking back through her medical history and he turned completely grey as the penny dropped. He sent us off for an MRI pretty quickly after that.

In his defence, a lot of doctors don't understand MS. Many haven't had to deal with it before and it's not the most straightforward disease to diagnose. I also reflect that in the time when I was born, you'd likely see the doctor who delivered you into the world but now, we tend to go to these large medical centres where you end up seeing a different doctor every time. The lack of continuity of care only makes it harder to get a handle on the real picture and I think the way we systemise our health in the modern world has a lot to answer for.

I was devastated at the news that Regina had MS. The only other person I knew with the condition was a lady who used to live around the corner from us when I was a kid. Her first noticeable symptom was that she started dragging her leg whilst walking. It started off that simply one day and the next thing I knew she became worse and worse until she died. I thought that would be Regina's fate.

I began to research the disease; the internet is wonderful! And I could see that there were things to be done and then we also contacted the MS Society and they were incredibly helpful. I was able to come around to believing that MS wouldn't be the death sentence I had in my mind. Really, my initial reaction was just ignorance.

Our attitude to how we wanted to live the rest of our life changed from that moment of diagnosis. We'd always just plodded along; working, paying the mortgage, simply meandering through life but now, we had something to live for. It became imperative to live as wholly and fully as possible while we could enjoy things.

One of the first things we did was buy a caravan so we could explore more of Australia. And that was fun for a bit but it fast became impractical so we sold it and used the money to take a trip to Vietnam. And Regina thrived on this trip. It was a fairly rigorous adventure that included lots of touring and climbing stairs to temples and other attractions. But people couldn't believe how well she powered along. She made the most of every opportunity, even if it meant us dragging her the last few steps to get to a temple. Her determination to experience everything was just so inspiring to us all. But she's always been a strong, determined woman and it's one of the things I love in her the most.

Being confronted by a disease such as MS forces you to reshuffle your priorities. It's no longer about having a lot of money for the sake of having money or working all the time to advance your career; instead it's about creating experiences where you can enjoy life together. And because your priorities turn to having a full and meaningful life while you can, you'll naturally find yourself redefining your financial or budgeting goals.

Money to me is not for saving or investing. It's simply for having a home, food and to enjoy and experience life. I'm not suggesting you throw caution to the wind, but I'm not as nervous about budgeting as I once was. I've already warned Jack that he'll probably have nothing by the time Regina and I keel over!

***

We told our son Jack immediately about Regina's diagnosis. Jack's one of those kids whose mind always jumps to the worst possible scenario. We could hear a weather forecast for bad storms and he'll immediately assume it's going to turn into a city-flattening cyclone. Given that, we realised we had to give him a lot of time and nurturing to get his mind around what was happening. The only thing he seemed concerned about initially was if his mum was going to die from the disease. Explaining a disease like MS is an enormous concept for a young kid to try and comprehend. I'm glad we had the materials and guidance from the MS Society so we could give Jack the information he needed to process what was going on.

But it's like anything in life. Your reaction to events is shaped by what you're exposed to and unfortunately Jack has been exposed to chronic illness at a young age. When I was nine – roughly the same age as Jack was when he found out about his mother – I had a brother who suffered a traumatic brain injury through a bike accident. I clearly remember the police coming to the door of our family home on Boxing Day and breaking the news to us and that event changed our whole life. A lot of things changed but certainly my parent's focus became my brother and from an early age I learned to be very independent. I reckon I basically raised myself.

My brother's injury has probably prepared me in some small way for what we're going through now. His situation was quite difficult to deal with and even though I learned to become quite independent I still felt abandoned for a long time because my parents gave their entire focus and attention to my brother. Our life was all about hospital visits or re-arranging our lives around him when he was home. And as horrible as it all sounds, those childhood experiences have educated me so as I don't make the same mistakes now with my own family.

I'm very vigilant as to Jack's experiences and ensuring he doesn't have the same childhood as I did. I try to protect him from the burden of illness as much as possible.

And I think I have a few more tools in my backpack than most in how to deal with illness in the family. I was so totally devastated at Regina's diagnosis but the consequences of it didn't hit me like a tonne of bricks as it would for most people because I'd already experienced a similar situation earlier in life.

But I do experience tremendous frustration that I can't fix something that is so important to me. I just want to eliminate the MS from Regina's body. I've spent my whole life looking after myself and those around me and suddenly this was one thing I couldn't fix. It's the man's job to fix things; it's what we do. It's an incredibly confronting and frustrating feeling. Regina never whinges about how poorly she's feeling either so it's hard for me to offer to make it better for her.

On the flip side, I don't feel like I can confide in her – let alone complain to her – when there's something going wrong in my life because I feel like my troubles are insignificant compared to hers. A few years ago I had to have my gall bladder removed and the pain was excruciating. I'd wander around the house at night in agony and Regina would be really concerned but I couldn't allow myself to let on how bad I felt. She now comes to the doctor with me whenever I have to go. It's her way of ensuring she knows the full story and I guess it's my way of informing her when I'm not well and I don't feel like I'm complaining directly to her. I might not tell her everything but I now realise she still picks up on a fair amount of it.

Just because I don't confide all my worries and pain to Regina doesn't mean I feel left behind. Frankly the happiness of my wife and son is a far greater priority.

**

Soon after Regina's diagnosis we had an occupational therapist visit our home and it was an entirely confronting and uncomfortable experience. The long list of modifications the therapist suggested we make was just jaw-dropping. We'd have to fit a lift, rip out any stairs, add handrails everywhere and refurbish the bathrooms. She basically wanted to turn our home into a hospital ward.

By the time the therapist had completed her assessment I was ready to strangle her. I got the feeling that she was putting Regina into a wheelchair before she even needed to be. I could tell Regina was becoming increasingly upset by everything she was hearing and I personally felt like we were being criticised and condemned for the way we lived.

The experience with the occupational therapist taught us a valuable lesson though. It taught us to contemplate where and who we got our advice from. It taught us that it was okay to ignore advice or dismiss information that didn't resonate with us.

I'm a fire fighter and my work mates serve as my extended family and those guys have been my biggest support network. In fact I find they're probably the people I turn to first for help and support. A few weeks ago I was interstate for a training exercise and Jack sustained an injury to his knee and Regina was finding it difficult to do everything she needed to for Jack. One text message to a colleague and they rallied around and divided the chores and it was just done. No hassle, not fuss, no guilt. It was very re-assuring. They know I'd do the same for them, but having that infallible support network is crucial. The camaraderie is a huge bonus in my job and I suspect the great majority of people don't have the same level of support in their work environment.

I think our experience with MS has also brought us closer together as a work crew. The team are constantly keeping an eye out for us, as well as each other, but they're also great at reminding me that it's not all about work and that looking after your family is far more important. They're very good at helping me put things into perspective. By that I mean recognising what needs to be prioritised and when not to sweat the small stuff. They also know when not to 'poke the bear....' We joke about it but they know on bad days my contribution to saving a life is that I don't kill someone!

When Regina spends any time in hospital, Jack and I are always inundated with people dropping off meals. I'm sure we fatten up quite a bit in those weeks, but people just want to help without intruding and one of the easiest ways they can think to help is by cooking. They want to be part of your support network without interfering. And admittedly I sometimes just want to deal with everything by myself but I've come to realise that people need that connection with you.

I'm fortunate that my work also provides for carer's leave and that's been a big bonus in being able to support Regina when things have been tough. I know a lot of other workplaces don't offer this and for us it's been a saviour. It's allowed me to find a great sense of balance and has certainly minimised pressure. I'm thankful that when I need to spend a day at home with my wife I'm able to make the decision and arrangements quickly and easily and it doesn't contribute any unnecessary stress in taking a day off from work.

My own roster is also ideal in that each week I work two days of ten hour shifts and two nights of 14 hour shifts. I'm only away two nights and I get quite a few days at home with Regina during the week as well. I've been really lucky to work a schedule like that but the advice I'd give someone else who needed to spend time at home looking after a loved one is to have the guts to go to your boss and try and work out a schedule that suits you both. There's always a compromise and people are often more accommodating than we give them credit for. Empathy can come from all sorts of surprising areas.

Life has also changed quite a bit since Regina recently gave up work. Due to my roster I used to spend a lot of days during the week by myself. As I mentioned, I've always been highly independent and I like my alone time. I don't have much time to myself any longer so it's been an adjustment. And I think it's important for anyone in a similar situation to ensure they find their own hobbies or carve out their own time so as they retain a sense of themselves. It's imperative to have an outlet. Couples would find the same situation in retirement but it's just another challenge that living with a chronic illness brings to your life that you never anticipate and you can never really prepare for.

I do worry now that Regina has stopped work she'll become socially isolated. She has started joining me and my work mates more when we go out for coffee, and that in itself has changed the dynamic, because now other wives come along too. It's actually been good for us, because when my colleagues and I would go out all we'd do was talk about work and then we'd go to work and talk about it some more. Having our wives and partners along means we're getting our heads out of work for a while, so it's had a positive effect.

My previous priorities in life were similar to most people, I guess. We wanted to work hard to pay off the mortgage, get Jack through school and have a bit of money in the bank for a rainy day. But now, our guiding principle is to just enjoy life and not sweat the small stuff. We now firmly understand that life is not a dress rehearsal. We're not sitting around practicing life....this is the only shot you get. And so easily a life-changing event can come along for anybody, at any time. And I used to be that person who sweated the small stuff and I'd become quite agro about things that went wrong. And it's that type of attitude that will fast lead you down the path of depression. I know. Now I've got the capability to step back and say 'so what? Who cares?' and move on.

I still have goals that motivate me, but the difference is that I've let go of the stuff that I can't fix and focus instead on the stuff that I can fix. And within the things that I can fix, there's still a process of prioritisation going on so as I work out the most important thing to tackle first and what really doesn't matter in the greater scheme of things.

Regina's own attitude to life has changed too. She rarely sweats the small stuff any longer. But I can see her frustration in not being able to do some of the things she used to be able to. I know she feels terrible that she's not contributing to the household income now that she's left work but it just doesn't faze me in the slightest. I want her to be healthy and safe and enjoying life – for the both of us. And besides, she's still the major contributor in how our house is run and our son is raised. Her job is vitally important.

In those first few years after the diagnosis, Regina tearfully confided to me a few times that she was worried she wouldn't be around to see Jack grow up. The longer we live with MS the more re-assured we feel that's not going to be the case and we certainly make the most of our time together. We both decided from the start that we wanted Jack to be able to adjust quickly and easily to change. And one of the ways we did that was by travelling and also moving house. And we may even move again if we find we want a change. I guess you could say we're encouraging a gypsy lifestyle!

Jack has also recently changed schools and is participating in an air force cadet's programme. We can both see how focussed and aspirational he has become for a career in the military and again, I know that peer support gives Regina a tremendous amount of faith that he's going to have a network similar to my own via his air force family. We've noticed that even at this young age, Jack and all his mates in the Cadet's watch out for one another.

Regina's diagnosis really was the moment the penny dropped for me that there is no dress rehearsal in life. And we're lucky that we're both very open and honest people who communicate easily. From the very start we could have some confronting and real conversations about how we were going to tackle this disease head on. And how you choose to manage expectations and solutions is going to be unique to everyone. For us, we wanted to travel and do the things that we might not be able to do very easily in ten years' time. We've had a few people infer to us that we were spending a lot of money on travel but in our mind we want to be able to enjoy life for as long and as much as possible while we can. I know Regina's not going to die from MS but her mobility is sadly declining and I want her to be able to experience as much of the world in comfort before things become too difficult. We fully realise you can still do quite a lot in life from a wheelchair but we're grabbing every opportunity we can before that becomes a permanent fixture.

I think some of the issues surrounding why people judge us for the way we're living our life come from the fact that MS is largely an invisible disease. They'll look at Regina and can't understand what's wrong with her. Only those very close to us understand the debili-tating fatigue and the struggle she has in walking any distance, but the other factor is that the MS is always changing. Her symptoms today may be vastly different next month. We call MS our little mystery basket! (MS = Mystery and Surprise). So again, we live in the moment. If people want to be ignorant as to how MS really effects someone, that's their problem, not ours.

I think Regina probably finds it frustrating to think that her work colleagues might not understand why she recently gave up work. She doesn't look sick and I'm sure many of them wouldn't understand the draining effect working every day was having on her health. And it wasn't just the physical fatigue but also the cognitive and emotional drain.

The group of friends we have now understand the cognitive fatigue Regina experiences. They never pressure her if she momentarily drops out of a conversation and understand that she's often happy to sit and listen and enjoy the company.

I try not to think about the future, preferring to take everything a day at a time. We've had to take it that way because the MS can be so wretchedly awful some days and quite stable others. And Regina is also the type of person who will keep pushing herself until she crumbles. But she always bounces back. We bought a wheelchair a while back. It just sits in the cupboard. Regina wants to get rid of it but I don't want to do that. I just don't know when or if we'll need it and in my mind if we do need it then it's one less problem I need to deal with immediately in sourcing a chair.

She's defiant and says "I'll never use it!" and my reply is always "Good! It can sit there and rot then, but Regina, I still want it there so I can help you as quickly and easily as possible if it comes to that."

She also wanted to convert one of our spare bedrooms, which meant getting rid of the bed in there. But again, I wanted to have that option of having a spare bedroom in case we needed to get someone over to provide home help or look after her if I was away. I was never trying to jump to the worst case scenario, but it was just my way of coping and knowing I was prepared if something happened. I don't sit there and dwell on the bad stuff, but I like feeling I've got some of the bases covered.

The thing about MS is that you don't just care for the person with MS but you also have to make sure you've got yourself organised. Personal organisation is a form of self-care. And you might have to take that in baby steps, but it is important. It is also no easy task to change your own habits and natural reactions to various events.

One of the most frustrating things about the role of a carer is that there is so little financial support or access to benefits, especially for someone in our situation where I'm still working. We have had to make some sacrifices and I don't think the government – any government – understand the burden placed on families living with a chronic illness. It's only small adjustments here and there, but it adds up to a very real financial impact. Regina would be the first to keep working if she could. I certainly want to keep working as long as possible, but I find myself having to take a lot of time off to help care for her. Private health cover is also another enormous expense but it does little to assist us in the treatments or providing the things Regina needs.

The craziest bit of advice we were given when we started investigating what benefits might be available was that we should get divorced. That's right, we'd be better off financially if we divorced because Regina could get a disability pension and I could get a single dad's benefit. It was mind blowing to have that suggested! Naturally we wouldn't even entertain the idea. I'd rather starve before we even considered doing that. But that's how crazy the welfare system is in Australia and I don't want to be one of the ones who rort it.

If I had to offer advice to anyone newly diagnosed it would be to understand as much about the disease and how it affects people as possible. It's important to recognise that MS can and will affect everyone differently, so people will naturally experience a wide range of emotions in living with it.

I've learned that just being there for Regina is enough sometimes. I don't have to say anything or figure out a solution, I just have to be there to support her.

On the flip side, I try to relate to the experience that Regina is going through. I guess it's called empathy. She used to hate giving herself injections and I always had to encourage her to take her medication, but one day I gave myself an injection just to see what it was like. And from that point on I realised why she hated them so much. It wasn't very pleasant at all. You can't always experience everything that your partner with MS is going through but there's definitely some experiences that are comparable and it's an important exercise to put yourself in their shoes.

I often say to Regina that if I could take her pain, even for just 24 hours, I would. She's my world so that seems the least I could do. But sadly I can't and I find that hugely frustrating.

But I wouldn't change anything about my life. I think my job in emergency services has conditioned me to deal with trauma and certainly growing up with a brother with a brain injury has. In emergency services we see some pretty awful stuff and we're also trained to deal with the worst case scenario, so I'm probably fairly pragmatic when it comes to how we need to get on with life. But none of that eliminates the frustration I feel for Regina's situation. That complete lack of control to be able to fix the MS or just make it go away and leave us alone.

I think so many of us live our life thinking we're bullet proof. We see bad things happen to other people but never entertain that it could happen to us. But I'm here to tell you it can and does happen to people just like us. And now knowing that bad stuff can happen to anyone has fortified me even more. I've seen first-hand that it can happen to anyone. I learned that through my brother's accident and now with my wife. If anything, it just empowers me to take greater control of the life we are living.

JACK BROOK – SON

"I really worry about Mum's future and I hate that not much is known about MS. But then I think that there's no point in worrying about something I can't control. I'd rather just live life now and worry about what's going to happen later."

My mum was diagnosed in 2010 when I was ten years old. I clearly remember that Mum and Dad came to pick me up from school and that was when they told me. I just fell apart. I don't think I really knew what MS was but I remember thinking it was a death note. I still get upset thinking about that moment.

We came home after school and we all sat down together and talked about what MS was and what it meant for Mum. The MS Society had sent an information pack to explain things about the disease. The pack included these great comics that made everything quite clear for me. And Mum and Dad were really great about everything and I felt like I was able to ask them questions.

I try to assist Mum in any way possible, whether it's just helping her get around or even doing as many chores around the house as I can. Mum has good days and bad. It's pretty easy to tell if she's on one of the bad days because she finds it hard to speak or walk.

Mum often gets frustrated with how the MS affects her. She bakes the most amazing cakes but sometimes when she's decorating them her hands won't work properly and she swears at the cakes. It makes her so mad. I try to help her and I really like cooking too.

But Mum can frustrate me at times too. She loves wearing her heels but she's such a gumby when she wears them and Dad will have to help her walk. I think Mum looks beautiful in heels but I always try to talk her out of wearing them because I don't want her to hurt herself walking.

Mum can get a bit emotional some times. The older I grow the more I understand why. She must really hate having MS. But when she's a bit sad, Dad and I are always around to try and make her laugh. I love being able to do that for my Mum. In fact, I think I use my sense of humour to make myself feel better as well.

The biggest thing I want other kids to know is that if their own Mum or Dad was diagnosed with MS they're not going to die from it. MS can be a pretty scary thing to try and figure out but knowing that it won't kill you helps. It might slow them down a bit but there's different grades of MS so it depends on which grade they are as to how bad things might be. I look at my Mum who's still making sure she lives her life every day as best she can and that helps me understand MS.

Only a few months after Mum and Dad told me about the MS we all went to New Zealand for a holiday. It was great for us all to be together and have fun. I think they wanted to travel as much as they could before the MS got too bad.

Living with a mum who has MS has taught me that you've got to live life to the fullest. I think about other kids who sit inside all day and play computer games and I think I'm lucky that I realise the value of life now and that you've got to enjoy things while you can.

I know I've had to grow up a bit faster than other kids my age. When Dad's at work I have to be the man of the house. I can't just sit back and let Mum do everything; I have to pitch in as well. I know I do a lot more cleaning and chores around the house than other kids my age. I reckon most kids would go straight home from school and play computer games but I make sure I come home and help Mum first. I only get to play my X-Box on a Friday night or sometimes in the school holidays. I must admit it's good when Dad's home because we can share the chores and I might get to play my X-Box more!

I really worry about Mum's future and I hate that not much is known about MS. But then I think that there's no point in worrying about something I can't control. I'd rather just live life now and worry about what's going to happen later.

People don't understand the silent pain that MS sufferers go through. When I try to explain to other people what MS is I say to them that just because Mum looks good on the outside, doesn't mean she's feeling very well on the inside. People don't always understand that someone can look really healthy but not be well at all. It's confusing to them.

Dear Brooky and Stink,

(My Men, My Protectors, My Heros, My World!)

This is a letter to you both to let you know how much I love and treasure you and how you both keep me wanting to fight the fight that is "My Life."

"Love you," "I love you," "Mmmm....mm," or "Left Shoe." Not a day goes by that these words, or sounds, aren't said between the three of us. But when these few words are uttered in a somewhat habitual way, what do they really mean? At least for me anyway....

Stink (aka Jack), I am bursting with pride whenever I look at you. You are a rare species, and no, I'm not talking about the fact that you are a Ranga. It's the fact that you are still happy to hold my hand when I need help…in public… I mean in complete view of other teenagers! This to me means more than you will ever know. You would have to be one of the very few 15 year olds who don't have the 6 meter 'stay away from me in public' zone that can only be infiltrated in times of hunger or low cash supplies.

It amazes me how you stay true to yourself and you don't buckle to peer group pressures. Is that because of stubbornness or just red hair? Whatever it is, harness it and learn to use it wisely. It will come in handy - trust me! You have your goals and you are working hard to achieve them. The sky's the limit for you so don't get stars in your eyes or become side tracked by watching the Comedy Festival's on TV. I laugh at your jokes because I am your mother and I love you. However, you know how you watch people singing on YouTube and you say "why doesn't someone tell them they can't sing?" Consider yourself told! You are a pilot…NOT a comedian. This is said with love, not sarcasm, and if I could, I would insert the emoji with a little face blowing a kiss.

Whatever the future holds for you, know that you have done your very best and I am so proud of you. I know you will keep striving until you get to where your heart aches to be. And for this - your dedication and determination - I adore you. Along the way there will be many ups and down, as you have already encountered. I worry about what life has in store for you but in hard times I have no doubt you will just pull yourself together and say your mantra 'shit happens…just deal with it' and do just that. At just 15 you have certainly calmed many a stressed moment, bringing me back down to reality with your wise and 'swear jar exempt' mantra.

Thank you. You are your father's son…except for the red undies!

Sorry Brooky… You didn't think I wouldn't bring up your biggest foible? I was sure Super Heroes wore red capes. Not mine. You choose to wear red undies, and for you I have been known to visit up to four major shopping centres in one day to purchase the aforementioned Super Powered items. This is how much I love you! It may be a good time to point out that these Super Powers are strictly emotional and by no means biological.

The things we have done in the 30 years we have been best friends….. Well good grief it's a wonder we're still in one piece! We survived the 80's with the streaked mullets and Material Girl fashions, Cold Chisel concerts and cheap wine out of plastic bags, only to be hit with hyper-coloured t-shirts in the 90's. What was with them and your little hissy fit when I "broke one" by seeing what would happen if I put it in the freezer? We've walked on fire, sung loudly, burped the alphabet, laughed hysterically and cried many tears. Our hearts have been hurt more times than I would like to count, but on each occasion we've been there for each other.

Then just when we thought we were on the home stretch this MS thing happened. I call it a thing because it really doesn't deserve a title of significance. Feed it and it will grow? Who knows! Ignore it and it might go away. Nope, not that either. But what I do know is the fact that on my darkest days you manage to make me laugh. Sometimes I could slap you for doing it because I just want to wallow in self-pity for a couple of minutes, but you know me better than myself. You know that I'm a better person than that and you pull me out of the hole that's consumed me. I worry about who is being strong for you. Who has your back, so to speak? I'm a heavy weight to bare, in more ways than one, and I just hope that you get things off your chest with our wonderful friends that we are lucky enough to have.

"What if?" We've been there and done that. Now it's time for the "what's next?" We just have to sit back and take one day at a time. And on the upside, at least life is never boring. We never know what we will be getting from one day to the next. Who needs stability at our age? Not you and me....My Super Hero, My Husband, My Protector, My World.

Mmmm mmm... for supporting me in anything I choose to do, even if it's to shave my head, grow out my grey hair and wear retro clothes.

Love you... for your understanding and even, not understanding.

Love you... for staying... when I gave the opportunity to leave.

Love you... for your constant struggle to accept that you can't fix me.

For this.....

"My left shoe." xxx

STEVE ROBERSTON - HUSBAND

"I can't comprehend what it's like to have the disease but I don't think Wenda can comprehend what it's like for me to NOT have the disease, but to still be affected by it every day."

Wenda and I met in 1998 at a Toastmaster's public speaking course. Wenda was already a toastmaster and I was at the workshop to improve my public speaking skills for work. Wenda was actually one of the event facilitators and during an earlier session I learned she was originally from the UK. I started to approach her as I wanted to chat about living and working there. But I never got the chance because she actually turned her back on me and started to walk away! I came to find out later she had turned away flustered because she actually liked me and thought she'd turn red with embarrassment. At the end of the event she asked me out for a drink anyway and as they say, that was that.

I remember our first 'official' date was weeks later on the 7th July. It's a bittersweet date to be honest as my sister passed away from breast cancer on that date in 2005. We dated for about 18 months, getting married in February 2001, so we've been married for 14 years now.

I was working as an engineer when we met and Wenda was doing post-doctoral research at the University of Queensland in Brisbane. She didn't have any symptoms of MS when we met, although she was diagnosed only a few months before we were married so we both suspect she'd been living with MS for a while prior to that.

She originally felt the onset of the symptoms when she was doing step aerobics. She explained to me that she would constantly feel as if she was losing her balance on the step equipment. Neither of us thought much of it at the time but then her feet started to go numb. She'd actually experienced this kind of numbness a few times before when she was completing her PhD.

When these minor symptoms happen you don't really chalk it up to much – certainly not a life-changing diagnosis. Your body does funny things when you're under stress and while life was great for us, we were planning a wedding, doing visa applications and Wenda was progressing in her career, so there was no shortage of major life events to contend with.

But when the numbness continued she finally went to her GP for a check-up, who then sent her to a neurologist. I really thought her doctor's check-up would reveal something as simple as a pinched nerve or a virus that she could just get a prescription for. Most people don't really go to the doctor thinking that it's ever going to be something that can't be solved easily.

Wenda still wasn't worried and went to that first neurology appointment by herself. But when she eventually left the clinic she was very upset and called to tell me the news. The neurologist had examined her and taking into account all the symptoms she'd described he felt certain she had MS. That night there was a lot of tears but Wenda's determined personality soon clicked in and she went into 'let's sort this out' mode. She booked in to see a psychologist the next day, got everything she needed to off her chest, had a few more tears and then crossed it off her list of things to do. She's just like that; she sorts stuff out.

I now know that her no-nonsense attitude was the way that Wenda needed to process what was going on. She needed to have a plan of attack as a way of dealing with the diagnosis piece-by-piece. For me, processing the diagnosis still continues 15 years later. It's still going on this day as you never really know what life is going to chuck at you and in the back of my mind, there is still an element of uncertainty with the disease and the course it will take.

After the neurologist had performed further tests and definitively confirmed MS, Wenda sat down with me and explained that she totally understood if I didn't want to proceed with the wedding. I knew a little bit about MS, having met a friend of her's who had been living with it for a number of years. But I certainly didn't know what caused MS, what the different diagnosing factors were, what we'd most likely have to manage or how the disease was treated. There was a lot of information to go through at the time and I'll be completely honest, I'm not the sort of person to sit down and read up on it all overnight. I looked upon the situation as having such uncertainty and also realised that MS can be different for each individual case anyway; I thought that if I was to prejudice my reaction to the disease with too much information early on it might not be the right path to take.

I'm sure Wenda found this incredibly frustrating, maybe perceiving me as not taking an active interest in the issue. But that wasn't the case. If I can't anticipate what's coming, I find it very difficult to prepare. And I find it doubly difficult if I try and anticipate something to then get it completely wrong and have to alter my plan of action yet again to compensate.

I guess you could describe my approach as reactive rather than contemplative but with such an unpredictable disease, that's really all I could do.

As an engineer I'm dealing with people as much as technical elements in my work. I'm of the firm belief that every problem we've got facing humanity at the moment, with money as no object, has a technical solution that can be implemented to achieve the desired outcome. But the moment you put the human factor into the mix, it will completely change the equation.

I reflect back on my 10 year university reunion and one of my lecturers asked me which course I found the most beneficial within the engineering syllabus. My answer was sociology. My lecturer answered with 'so you've finally worked out what engineering is all about then!' In its very base form engineering is the application of a technical solution to a social context. But if you don't understand the social context then you've got no hope of delivering the right solution.

And I guess I approach a lot of things in life like this. You've got to mould and shape a solution to a particular situation and when you're dealing with human problems it's always different and always changing.

Having the conversation about whether we should continue planning for our life together was very surreal. I may have been naive but I simply took the approach that this was all just going to be one big journey and I loved Wenda so I was glad I was the one taking the journey with her. I never knew what that destination was going to be and I daresay Wenda didn't either. At the time, I didn't think about Wenda's diagnosis in terms other than the collective 'us.' It was 'us' on the journey and how would 'we' deal with this? And certainly for the first few years there was no change to the 'us' and it was only when her mobility started to become affected - along with peripheral numbness and the fatigue setting in - that I started feeling a resent-ment. I resented the disease when I reflected on what our life could have been like and now realised that we would be living it differently.

When you're relatively young, perhaps working on furthering your career and newly married, you sit back and imagine that in the very near future you'll be exploring the world, setting out on great adventures, buying houses, starting a family and building the great Australian dream. But as the MS started eddying in on Wenda's life all I could think was 'oh crap, we're going to need to factor in other things here.'

For most people, the event of changing career or having a child were things they had control over. But suddenly we were faced with something that we had very little control over. It's as if some divine power had pulled the carpet out from us and was explaining that certain options were no longer available. Sometimes I almost felt like it was a form of discrimination. Wenda and I weren't actively being discriminated against, but the sort of circumstances that were arising made it feel that way, in the choices that were denied us.

So yes, there was certainly resentment in those early days and a lot of uncertainty around the things we wanted to do as a married couple, such as travelling or having a family. I'll admit that I can be a 'glass half empty' type of guy at times and I struggled to positively contemplate our future life together.

And some 15 years later there's been no turning point for me as such, where I have experienced a jump in outlook or the dynamic of how I deal with things. Some days I'll realise I'm mentally annoyed by the impact that MS has on our family but I'm resigned to the fact that there's nothing to be done about it. Other days I'll take pleasure in the great things we can still do together. Sliding between the two different mindsets can be a frustrating thing to live with.

We both live with MS but we see it from two different angles; it's actually one of the most difficult things in our relationship. I can't comprehend what it's like to have the disease but I don't think Wenda can comprehend what it's like to not have the disease, but to still be affected by it every day. I think that's probably the hardest thing for me to live with. I guess you could say she's numb to the impact of MS on me.

We were blessed that we were eventually able to have a daughter. Wenda spent a while adjusting her MS treatment so she could try to get pregnant and we even tried IVF. But when we were unsuccessful in our attempts we sort of gave up and chose to move to the UK for a while instead. I think we both needed to regroup and distance ourselves from the exercise. When we returned from the UK, Wenda's MS seemed to be stable for the first year or two so we decided to roll the dice one more time. And as luck and fate would have it we were able to conceive this time.

But as we went through that process of trying to conceive I always had it in the back of my mind that I didn't know how I'd cope if Wenda's symptoms became worse and we were trying to raise a child whilst I was also working full time. I don't think I ever got my mind around this quandary and I know I wasn't overly supportive of Wenda during her pregnancy and our daughter's early years.

I was looking at the glass as being half empty and I tended to bury myself in work a bit to escape my thoughts and uncertainty. When I look back it was probably one of the hardest times I went through and if I had to relive the situation I know I'd be a little more positive, but at the time I just couldn't imagine how I was going to cope with everything. It was quite a narcissistic approach but I just let the negative thoughts escape and things snowballed.

That experience has taught me not to let the glass half empty thoughts prevail and what I'm trying to do – although I haven't quite mastered it yet – is to express my support through actions of patience instead. I think I took this approach because I realised that my negative thoughts reveal themselves in either frustration or anger; whereas if you can turn it around and channel the energy into patience then you'll pop out the other end of any adverse situation a lot better off.

One thing that living with someone with MS has done is reduced my level of tolerance for what I consider to be minor annoyances at work. To be honest, one of the things that ticks me off the most is when people complain about the things that seem to be a huge blight on their life, yet in reality those things are reasonably insignificant and they have complete control over being able to change them. Take for example the equity debate, which often seems to get championed by people that have control over and very real options and choices to have a full and satisfying career. I question whether the motivation of these champions is actually derived from a genuine desire for equity in its truest form or a pecuniary interest arising from perceived injustices.

But my wife has a disease with no cure and that limits the choices that we can make. I'm not saying that we can't have children or my own career path is limited, but living with MS certainly complicates not only the present but also the future. We're constantly dealing with elements of uncertainty. Where's the equality in that? We didn't ask for this disease. As far as we know we didn't do anything to bring it on ourselves and yet we're the ones who need to re-engineer our life to cope with it. Griping about inequality if you are in a position to shape your future through personal choices, sounds pretty silly to me when I think in those terms.

You want to know what real inequality feels like? It's not being able to function equitably in society as a whole and being treated as a different class of citizen. It's particularly galling being placed in that position by something that you cannot influence, that you didn't ask for nor do you have the ability to change. That's inequality. And unfair.

I'm incredibly lucky that my circle of friends are very supportive and understanding. They all have their own dramas in life too, so I guess our collective empathy towards each other helps us support one another.

My parents are the most generous and caring people you'd ever meet but I get frustrated with them occasionally because I feel they don't deal with some of the pressing issues at hand. Deep down I think it's the way they cope with the grief and pain of losing my sister. And truthfully, I can understand why they are the way they are. In some ways, it probably results in me not actively asking for them to give us any support in living with MS. I figure they have enough of their own things to deal with without dealing with our problems too. But in their defence, I've never worked out what I need from them either and they do ask what they can do to help. I guess I don't know what type of help to ask for.

My own support network is made up of a close circle of friends. They are sensitive when required and it's great to be able to talk to them when I need to. But in terms of day-to-day help we never really leverage off the support of others. Again, I'm not really inclined to ever ask for help; it's just not in my nature to do so. There are instances when I've said to people - be it friends or work colleagues - that the best thing they can give me is time. Time is a very valuable commodity for me. I actually think one of the best gifts you could give someone looking after a chronically ill person is time away from commitments or simply time to go out and take a moment for themselves. I wouldn't consider it escapism. I think it comes back to that notion of control. If you're given a chunk of time to spend how you wish, you have complete discretion over what you do with it. It's very liberating.

It's amusing when I talk to other people at work about what our normal family routine is. I'll explain that I get up in the morning and the first thing I'll do is take the dogs for a walk. That's a chore but it is a really nice way to start the day too. Then I'll help my daughter get ready for school. Then it's out the door for me and I'll work from 8am through to about 5.30pm or so before heading back home again. Most nights I'll cook and then get my daughter ready for bed, reading her a story before tucking her in for the night. After that I'll try to steal half an hour or so for myself and check the footy news or similar before doing a bit of tidying up around the house. Depending on what projects we've got going on at work I may even need to do a few more hours of work from home before hitting bed. Most nights I fall into bed completely shattered knowing that the next day is going to be absolutely the same.

When Wenda is feeling up to it she does a great job at helping with the workload, especially on the days when our daughter isn't attending school, but it's a relatively consistent routine and it's something we've fallen into an easy pattern with over the years. Given Wenda's lack of stability and mobility I prefer to take on as many of the kitchen duties as possible because I don't want her hurting herself in the kitchen. I don't actually mind cooking but the thing I struggle with the most is having to think about what it is I'm meant to be cooking whilst I'm cooking it. I like a bit of planning in that regard but I'm happy to relinquish the control of that planning to someone else. And I guess that's one of the best ways Wenda can lighten my own workload - by helping with that process. She's well aware of my dislike of the planning as we've talked about it on numerous occasions!

However, one of the things I struggle the most in supporting Wenda is providing the emotional feedback she needs. I know this might sound strange but I guess we're on different ends of the spectrum in what we need and how we express ourselves emotionally. When I'm confronted by situations that could potentially hurt me, I tend to withdraw. And that may well be a male thing.

But Wenda is the complete opposite and loves the hugs and all of that. So the emotional support that she needs doesn't come naturally or spontaneously from me. Instead it's something I find myself very consciously contemplating before delivering. Our different needs and provision of emotional support is something that can often spiral into discord if Wenda doesn't feel I'm tuned in. To be honest, it's something we bicker about a bit, and I love my wife dearly but we're just wired differently with respect to this.

I've often wondered if we took MS out of the equation if I'd react differently. I think that I should be providing stronger emotional support because of the MS. Unfortunately the MS will never go away so in my mind, there is a constant need to provide emotional support. And that's a big responsibility. It's a constant allocation of energy. I know that might sound uncaring and clinical but it's the reality of the situation.

When Wenda was first diagnosed we went to the MS Society and the psychologist we spoke to likened MS to a jar of jellybeans.

"You can take a jellybean out," he explained, "but the problem is that once the jellybeans are gone, you are done. And with MS it takes a lot more to put the jellybeans back in and with the progression of the disease, you might not get the jellybeans back to the same level. So you're constantly working with deficits in the form of decreasing energy – be it physical, mental or emotional."

I find myself in the fortunate position that I can top the jellybeans back up at the same rate as which I take them out, but the reserves do get drawn down again pretty quickly, so you can understand my own emotional fatigue. When you get to an energy level where by your personality is not able to be modified by your behaviour, your real personality comes to the surface; and it just happens that my natural personality is to be introverted.

And to be honest, I find that the only way I can top up my own jellybean jar of emotional energy is to withdraw somewhat. And if you've constantly got the disease in your face – and all of the other things that it brings – then you don't get the opportunity as frequently as you'd like to be able to do what you need to do to top up your reserves.

On reflection I believe that our marriage has actually become a lot stronger because of what we have to do to live with MS. It might sound like we're on tenterhooks all the time but I'm completely vested in always bouncing back from whatever it is we have to face each day. And part of the challenge in living with someone with MS is recognising that they can't always wait for that bounce back to occur. It's always going to be a delicate balance between providing what your partner needs and ensuring you're also looking after your own emotional needs. And even relationships free of chronic illness will operate in a similar way; but a chronic illness exerts a lot more pressure on time.

And I certainly don't have all the answers; all I can suggest is doing everything you can to figure out what works for you personally so that you never let the jellybean supply get critically drawn down. And I reckon that will need to be a constantly evolving strategy.

From my perspective, one of the most important coping mechanisms is being able to find time for yourself and to have the opportunity to do something you enjoy at your election. You need to have something you feel you're in control of – whatever that might be - it doesn't matter. I just know that you need to have something in your life that you know you can take control of. For me it's taking a few hours every week to play basketball with a team. For someone else it might be sitting on the sofa for an hour Googling pictures of dolphins. It's all about having that opportunity to escape and just be part of something away from the MS.

I don't know that humans, and particularly males, are inherently blessed with an emotional EQ to be able to cope with chronic illness. Let's face it….. It's all a pretty unnatural experience to go through. As males we'll always want to sit there and fix stuff but you just can't. So instead I think the important thing is to be able to maintain the personal energy supply so that you, in turn, can provide the emotional and physical support your partner needs.

We don't spend all our time wrapped up and talking about multiple sclerosis. Certainly we did for a while after Wenda was first diagnosed, but we were both trying to process what was happening. It rarely enters into the conversation much any longer. I guess over time you find a new sense of normal. It's understandable that you may feel engulfed and even swamped by MS in those first few years, but gradually you do stop focussing on the topic and other things start to become important – or at least more interesting – again. We spent the first couple of years on a quest for knowledge so we could try to take some semblance of control over how we were going to kick this thing in the butt. We wanted to be the exception to the rule. You do everything in your power to enhance your knowledge as quickly and as completely as possible. But I think it's also important to remember that no matter how knowledgeable you are about a chronic illness, it does tend to be an ever-changing scenario so you have to remain flexible and open to new ideas or situations. But even in those micro-adjustments you're still always learning. You're always trying to pick up as much information as you can.

I don't see much point in dwelling on all the miniscule details of MS once you've been living with the disease for a long time. You kind of get your processes in place and you work out how to cope with different things and that's just the way it is. After a decade of living with the disease I never find myself or Wenda sitting down and thinking about MS endlessly or being particularly reflective of why and how we do things. We just put one foot in front of the other and get on with life.

And that's not to suggest we're in denial or ignoring the MS.

It's always there but once you've talked about it quite a bit over the first few years there's really not much else to say about it. Naturally certain situations arise where we need to address how we'll deal with something, but I think by and large it's a case that once you've finally got your mind around how to live with MS you've drawn the line in the sand and you just get on with things.

Something that has really worked in our favour is that Wenda just won't give up. She never has since Day One. And to be honest, there's times when that defiant yet courageous attitude has placed strains and stresses on our life but I'm so proud she wants to keep throwing herself into life and do things that others may not even attempt if they were in a similar situation. Patience is not one of my wife's strong character traits!

Wenda and I look forward tremendously to watching our daughter grow up and turn into a wonderful and beautiful little girl. I think the things we've had to endure with MS have contributed to our daughter's character in such a way that she shows a level of empathy way beyond her years.

Wenda's condition has also given me pause to think about what makes me happy, especially in terms of my career. I'm making work decisions based on what makes me happy - and that's a positive thing to reflect on. Because if I can be happier at work I'll certainly be happier at home.

And I'm hoping that Wenda might be able to go back into the workforce at some stage in the future. I want her to feel that she's contributing to her own self-development and also the community.

There's been times when I've sat there and thought "I've had enough of MS; I want out." And I reckon Wenda would have similar thoughts at times. It's not that we want out from the relationship, but just to have the experience of 'normal' again. You've got to be able to separate those feelings of wanting to distance yourself from the disease, but not necessarily the person.

I've had to get my mind around the fact that the journey that Wenda goes on with MS does not have to be the same journey I take with it. We're both different personalities so it's only natural we'll process things differently, have distinct needs and certainly different ways of reacting to events. In the future we will probably both end up in the same place on our journey with MS, but we're both going to experience different ways of getting to that point. It's all just part of that continual learning process.

Dear Steve

I still remember your face when I told you I'd been diagnosed with MS. We just cried in each other's arms, thinking that our hopes and dreams of the future would never happen. The diagnosis was only 3 months before our wedding. At the time I couldn't help but think I was going to end up in a wheelchair and I was very serious about giving you the option of leaving. I wouldn't have held it against you. You simply looked at me in surprise and said nothing was going to change – you still wanted to marry me. I sometimes wonder that if you knew what you know now, would your answer still be the same?

I know I'm very lucky to have you as my husband. Not only are you a great Dad but you are a wonderful husband. Sometimes after a full day at work, you'll come home and cook dinner and bath our daughter. How does that make me feel? Most importantly grateful, but also frustrated and lazy! For example I may think 'if I hadn't gone to work, exercised or met a friend for coffee, would I have the energy to be a better wife?' One thing I've learned in living with MS is that I have to keep my mental and physi-cal health in check to preserve some quality of life. Having said that, it's extremely important that you – as my primary support network – maintain your own sense of work/life balance. I know how hard you work during the day as an engineer, and then you come home at night and continue working to keep the household running smoothly.

After some emotional discussions over the years, I think we are gradually becoming a pretty successful team. We're definitely planning to have more fun as a family; enjoy some adventures with our daughter - as she's growing up so fast - and go on some date nights to remember that we're husband and wife first, before we're carer and patient.

So my message to you is: "words cannot adequately express my appreciation for all you do and my love for you (even when you call me Gumby). Let's continue to have the same hopes and dream the same dreams, because I'm determined MS will not stop our plans."

Love Wenda

NANCY CLOAKE - GRAND DAUGHTER

"Grandma's condition ultimately inspired my career in research and more specifically within the areas of the brain and the immune system. Many patients with MS, their carers and families know there are researchers dedicated to finding the cure for MS. But many would not know our motivation and our passion to solve the puzzle."

I grew up on a farm in Forbes along with my younger brother and sister. It was a fairly normal and peaceful place to grow up and I think I probably had an upbringing much like any other Aussie kid – except that I knew my grandmother was disabled. My mother was 15 when grandma had a nasty fall at the hospital where she was working. Mum seems to remember that while it took a few years for the doctors to diagnose that grandma had MS, it was not long after the fall that she progressed into a wheelchair. Eventually my grandfather ended up leaving his job to look after grandma full time. Mum said in those early days they would take her to a lot of physio and hydrotherapy to help with rehabilitation; despite these efforts she continued to become worse. Back then in the late 70's there really wasn't the type of medications or drug therapies for MS that there are today.

As kids we would visit my grandparents a few times a year at their place in Macksville on the northern New South Wales coast. We were country kids so the beach getaways were always a lot of fun. By this stage, grandma had been living with MS for at least 15 years and

I'd never known her to be any other way. It wasn't like I looked at her and thought 'Oh, you have MS.' I just knew she was disabled and in a wheelchair but she was still my grandmother and I think that thought alone overrode anything else I might have thought.

I have vivid memories of doing the MS Read-a-thon when I was younger and also the 40 Hour Famine. But at that young age you participate in these campaigns and it's great to raise funds but I don't think I really had any keen perception of what I was specifically fundraising for or how it would help. With Mum's coaching I realised that my efforts in the MS Read-a-thon were helping grandma but still at that point I was quite blurry as to what MS actually was. In fact, I'm pretty sure even Mum had a hard time understanding what the disease entailed. All we knew and could see was that she was in a wheelchair and it affected her mobility, but we didn't know what other symptoms she might be experiencing.

It wasn't until many years later that I realised people could be diagnosed with MS but stay mobile for quite some time. I now understand how difficult it would have been finding any information about the disease back then but it would have been even more difficult if you were living in a rural area.

I always liked science at high school and part of me wanted to study medicine but I elected to do a degree in science instead. I attended the Charles Sturt University at Wagga Wagga where I graduated with a double degree in biotechnology and medical science. I had a keen interest in the anatomy of the brain and how the brain worked. In conjunction with this I was fascinated by how the immune system functioned and how in some situations it could break down and destroy your own body. Those two topics brought together my interest in MS. On top of this I had the family knowledge of MS via my grandma's experience.

As part of my undergraduate degree I studied an elective of clinical physiology and that led me to learn how to perform assessment tests for breathing, the heart and the brain using an EEG and ECG machine. I ended up working at the hospital in Wagga

Wagga assisting with EEG testing. And while I enjoyed the one-on-one interaction with the patients when I was taking the recordings, I realised the level I was training at through my degree wouldn't ever allow me to go any higher than what I was already doing. Ultimately it was this part-time work in the hospital that helped me decide the direction I wanted to take my career in science. I wanted to become the person who analysed the results and wrote the reports. I didn't want to remain a technician all my life; I just wanted more from my career.

By the middle of my third year I realised what I actually wanted to use my degree for. I was doing work experience at a lab in Brisbane and had the opportunity to work alongside medical research scientists . Working in the laboratory environment excited me. I was fascinated by how someone could take a question or problem and try to solve it scientifically. A few weeks in the lab and I was hooked! I wanted to be a researcher. It might have something to do with the fact that I've always loved solving puzzles.

I had to undertake a research project in the final year of my undergraduate degree and after my experience at the lab working in immunology - combined with studying it at university - I focussed my project on MS and how it's diagnosed and the current treatments; the only person I knew at the time with MS was my grandmother. I didn't have any connections to MS outside of her. But it was from this point that I realised researching MS brought all my interests together and that the personal connection I had to MS via my grandma couldn't be ignored. If I could make a difference in this particular area it would fulfil all my personal goals.

After I graduated in 2008 I decided to move up to Brisbane. I had met a guy during my earlier work experience stint (who would later become my husband) but I also wanted to complete a year of honours. I investigated who was heading up MS research projects in Brisbane and came across Dr Judith Greer. She was focusing on diseases that affected the nervous system, particularly those in which the immune response may play a role. The major focus of her lab was multiple sclerosis. Dr Greer was also the Postgraduate Coordinator for the Central Clinical Division of the School of Medicine for the University of Queensland, and with her help I successfully applied for an honours program at UQ under her direction. I later completed my doctorate with her lab, studying myelin protein gene mutation in MS.

As a kid I loved puzzle books and even to this day I always have a puzzle on my bedside table. Going into research where someone might pose a question to me on how to solve something or being able to recognise where the gaps are in research findings feeds my puzzle solving side. I find it tremendously fascinating to be able to pose a question, think through what you're doing and realise that you may be one of the first people to think in a certain way to solve a problem. It's exciting to think that as you set out to perform an experiment you might end up knowing the answers – or at least part of the answer – and be able to tell that to the world.

I remember when I was reading a lot of research papers for my undergraduate project I came across papers by Dr Greer and also Professor Michael Pender. And then a few years later when I undertook my own honours programme and eventually the PhD research, I was fortunate enough to meet and work alongside these scientists. When you're a student you think these type of people are unreachable; they're so far up on the podium as far as what I could hope to accomplish. And while meeting them both was a career highlight, I also realise that they're just like me. They want to solve puzzles.

My PhD was split across two parts. One part focused on finding an immune modulating treatment for relapsing remitting MS and the other area, which was a bit unexpected, was proteomics (the study of proteins) and their mutations within the nervous system. We wanted to explore how those mutations might affect the health of the cells in the brain that make the myelin coating on nerve cells, the substance that is damaged in MS.

As researchers we have to contend with the notion that any

research we start (or puzzles we try to solve) may not necessarily be concluded definitively. But that research still contributes to a greater pool of knowledge that another scientist may pick up a decade from now and continue on with, perhaps even finding the answers in a different way or finding answers to a different puzzle altogether.

As humans we're not here forever and no one ever has all the answers, so I can only consider it encouraging – rather than frustrating – that someone else might crack the puzzle before I do. You simply have to be happy that someone might take the work you've done and build on it. If we didn't think this way, no one would ever publish their findings! In fact, once you've published your findings you've essentially given other scientists the right to take your material and play with it. You've provided the hypothesis, the means and methods – a roadmap as such. And in fact, if your research couldn't be reproduced then no one could trust that it was real.

I think when it comes to the cure of MS there's still so much we don't understand surrounding the cause of the disease. I think it's widely accepted in scientific fields that the cause can be quite different in each person. There may well be sub-groups, where the cause is the same amongst a group of people, but one of the factors we're hoping to determine is if these various subgroups do in fact exist.

The immune system is very interesting because one minute it can be functioning well and the next moment it can go haywire. It is a system where the cells involved have a very high turnover because they're built to live long enough to fight off the problem presented, only to leave or die when their job is done. Sometimes they might leave a few cells remaining as a 'reminder' of what happened so if the problem occurs again, the cells know how to fight it.

But then a situation might occur where the cells are tricked (or don't remember how to fight the problem correctly) and auto-immune disease can occur. And when cells start moving down a path they weren't designed to help, it can be difficult to reverse the effect.

Pursuing a career in research is not for the faint-of-heart. You absolutely need to be passionate and dedicated to solving your chosen puzzle. Tenacity and strength are also required to take the critical feedback we often receive on our research. But also the constant battle for funds to be able to continue what we start. It might seem obvious to state, but research funds also fund our salaries, and when we're often battling for every cent just to fund the project itself, there's not a lot left over. I wouldn't say there's a tremendous feeling of financial security in being a researcher.

And before any of the research can even happen, we'll spend months (and sometimes years) refining our research grant applications and then waiting for a response, with no guarantee of success. I know many scientists will use that waiting time as an opportunity to begin their research just to find some preliminary conclusions in case they need to provide rebuttal material in response to a grant committee. They basically have to assume a certain amount of risk before the formal study even begins.

I do regret that I wasn't able to have a close relationship with my grandma because the MS was so progressed for her by the time I was old enough to enjoy her company. But the older she got, the more she'd sleep and less she'd talk. The disease really took a hold of her. As a young mother now I'm really aware of making sure my daughter gets to know her grandparents. I don't want her to have the same regrets I've experienced.

Grandma's condition ultimately inspired my career in research and more specifically within the areas of the brain and immune system. Many patients with MS, their carers and families know there are researchers dedicated to finding the cure for MS. But many would not know our motivation and our passion to solve the puzzle.

A brief history of MS research and diagnostic techniques

It is thought that multiple sclerosis was first recognised as a disease a little over 150 years ago. Augustus d'Este, the grandson of England's King George III, is now thought to have had MS based on a diary he kept until his death in 1848, in which he described having symptoms that sound much like MS, including blurred vision, weakness and numbness in his limbs, tremors and nocturnal spasms.

Twenty years after d'Este's death, the Parisian neurologist Jean-Martin Charcot was the first to identify and name MS. A female patient of Charcot's suffered from tremors, slurred speech and abnormal eye movements. He attempted to treat her, but to no avail. After her death, Charcot examined the patient's brain and discovered the tell-tale plaques of MS — the hardened scar tissue around nerve fibers. Though he is credited with the discovery of MS, Charcot thought the condition was rare.

In the latter half of the 19th century, examinations of MS symptoms began to be published — first by Dr. William Moxon in England in 1873, and then by Dr. Edward Seguin in the United States in 1878. Much of the observations these doctors made then are familiar to us today, including that MS is more common in women and that symptoms can differ from patient to patient. But because doctors were not yet knowledgeable of the body's immune system, MS couldn't yet be identified as an autoimmune disease.

In the early 1900s, researchers discovered chemicals that allowed them to observe nerve cells under a microscope. In 1916, James Dawson, a doctor in Scotland, described the inflammation and damage to myelin he saw when he looked at brain cells from people with MS under a microscope. The cells that make myelin — oligodendrocytes — were identified in 1928; later in 1943 research-ers then identified the composition of myelin.

In the 1960s, researchers discovered that MS is an autoimmune disease, one in which the body thinks it's being invaded and so attacks itself. This discovery led to the first trial of a potential therapy, the anti-inflammatory and immune-suppressing hormone ACTH, or adrenocorticotropic hormone.

The development of imaging techniques in the 1970s further advanced knowledge of MS. The first CAT scans, a circular array of X-rays, were performed on people with MS in 1978. CAT scans and magnetic resonance imaging (MRI), also developed during the 1970s, enabled researchers to see the brain in greater detail and thus develop better MS therapies.

The diagnosis of MS was further improved with the introduction of brain wave tests called "evoked potentials" which measure nerve conduction throughout the optic nerves, brain and spinal cord and often detect hidden areas of scarring and damage.

Despite these great strides in MS research and diagnosis, it wasn't until access to MRI machines became more widely available in the 1990s that huge changes were seen in the landscape of MS diagnosis. Many of the decade's advances sprang from the incredible power of new technology. Sophisticated techniques added to the MRI process allowed it to detect MS plaques earlier and more accurately than ever. That led to more rapid diagnosis of the disease. In 1970, the average time from a person's first symptom of MS until a definite diagnosis was seven years, but use of MRI technology reduced the time to six months. Now the plaque that causes symptoms can often be seen immediately. The power of a rapid, painless MRI scan to provide information is an incalculable blessing for doctors and patients alike.

ACKNOWLEDGEMENTS

I can say first and foremost that my family have been my 'everything.' My Mum and my Dad have suffered unbelievable pain throughout my diagnosis of both MS and then breast cancer and they held it together for me. They have supported and encouraged me to develop this book series and helped me believe in myself even when I wasn't so sure. My sister Rachel, also a journalist, offered endless support and suggestions and never once let me down. Her ideas have made this a stronger concept.

A huge thanks to each and every person I interviewed for this book; for laying your souls bare and trusting me with your story. Stephanie, Emma, Paul, Louise, Karen, Helen, Jay, Ratu, Adam, Ian, Jack, Steve and Nancy… you will be friends for life and I thank you for the strength and inspiration you have all given me. I truly believe the journey you have shared will make a tremendous impact on the lives of others.

And similarly, to the family members who were the subject of the interviews. I know how confronting it is to read about yourself and in many cases, read about issues or emotions you had no idea about. In some cases it may have opened a deep-seated wound but know that at their very heart, these are stories of love.

To Ebony Cavallaro for taking on the challenge of interviewing my four friends for this book. You were thoughtful, well-researched, and empathetic yet probing in your interview and I feel honoured that you have been able to contribute to such an important part of this book.

To Mandy Lee and Zoe Chapman at MS Research Australia for their wonderful guidance in contacting additional people to interview for this book. I have loved getting to know you both and can't wait for a fabulous year ahead working on the Kiss Goodbye to MS campaign.

To Tim Ferguson. My dear friend, whose advice in writing the first book has stuck with me ever since and irrevocably changed the course of my life. You have shown me that while MS is indeed a game changer, that in devoting my (precious) energy to something I love, I will always be able to push through the difficult days. You have taught me that everything matters now (remember the le Carre quote "There's nothing so dangerous as a spy in a hurry".....) In writing the books as I do now, I have never been happier. I can't wait for the next project to unfold.

***

If you enjoyed this book you may be interested
in the other two books in the series.

Taking Control - is the inspiring journey through the lives of 15
people living with MS. Read how they were diagnosed and address
their greatest fears to go on and create a new life. *(Available now)*

Book 3 will curate the knowledge of MS Nurses from
around the world. Their unique insight into dealing and living
with MS will provide valuable information to
patients and families alike. *(Coming soon)*

Buy online at www.take20stories.com